# THE SUPER EASY KETO DIET COOKBOOK

*575 Best Keto Diet Recipes of All Time (30-Day Meal Plan to Lose Weight and Wellness)*

~ *Rachel Collins*

# Copyright © 2019 by Rachel Collins

All rights reserved. No part of this publication may be reproduced, distributed, or transmitted in any form or by any means, including photocopying, recording, or other electronic or mechanical methods, without the prior written permission of the publisher, except in the case of brief quotations embodied in critical reviews and certain other non-commercial uses permitted by copyright law.

Limit of liability/Disclaimer of Warranty: The publisher and the author make no representations or warranties with respect to the accuracy or completeness of the contents of this work and specifically disclaim all warranties, including without limitation warranties of fitness for a particular purpose. No warranty may be created or extended by sales or promotional materials. The advice and strategies contained herein may not be suitable for every situation. This work is sold with the understanding that the author is not engaged in rendering medical, legal or other professional advice or services. If professional assistance is required, the services of a competent professional person should be sought. Neither the publisher nor the author shall be liable for damages arising herefrom. The fact that an individual, organization, or website is referred to in this work as a citation and/or potential source of further information does not mean that the author or the publisher endorses the information the individual, organization, or website may provide or recommendations they/it may make.

Photography © 2019 Stockfood/Benjamin Cohen, Stockfood/Giada Harper, Despositphotos.com, Stockfood/Jeff Walker, Stocksy/Sarah Remington, Stocksy/Sarah Bista, Stockfood/Harald Wasserman, Shutterstock.com, Stockfood/Kimberly White, Shutterstock.com

Illustrations © James Foster

Cover design by Neil Bercow

# **_Dedication_**

*To John and the kids,*

*You inspire me not only in the kitchen, but in every part of life. I love to cook, in no small part, because of the excitement and appreciation you have shown for my home-cooked meals all along the way. Our time together in the kitchen and the countless hours we have spent around the table are my favorite memories of all.*

*To dark chocolate,*

*my companion through many a long night of writing.*

*To you (yes, you)!*

# TABLE OF CONTENTS

## FOODS FOR KETO DIET   1

## 30-DAY MEAL PLAN & SHOPPING LIST   4

### CHAPTER 1
13   SMOOTHIES & BREAKFAST

### CHAPTER 2
36   SOUPS & SALADS

### CHAPTER 3
62   BEEF & LAMB

### CHAPTER 4
88   PORK

### CHAPTER 5
114   POULTRY

### CHAPTER 6
143   APPETIZERS & SNACKS

### CHAPTER 7
FISH & SEAFOOD   167

### CHAPTER 8
VEGGIES & SIDES   192

### CHAPTER 9
DESSERTS & DRINKS   217

### CHAPTER 10
DRESSINGS, SAUCES & SEASONING   238

### CHAPTER 11
GLUTEN & DAIRY-FREE, VEGAN   260

## MEASUREMENT CONVERSION CHARTS   270

## ABOUT THE AUTHOR   273

## RECIPE INDEX   274

# Foods for Keto Diet

## Foods which are allowed

The following foods are viewed as the best for the keto diet plan. They are impressively low on carbs. These include:

- Dairy products like hard cheese, soft cheese, whipping cream, butter, cream cheese, Greek yogurt, cottage cheese, and sour cream.
- Meat and poultry should be preferably grass-fed and organic.
- Fish/Seafood - Preferably eating anything that is caught wild like catfish, cod, flounder, halibut, mackerel, mahi-mahi, salmon, snapper, trout, and tuna
- Above ground veggies like cauliflower, broccoli, and zucchini and etc.
- Leafy green vegetables like spinach, kale, and etc.
- Seeds and nuts like almonds, pumpkin seeds, sunflower seeds, pecans, walnuts, chia seeds, Brazil nuts, cashews, and pistachios, etc.
- Berries like blackberries, raspberries and other effect berries which are low glycemic in nature.
- Avocados
- Sweeteners like erythritol, stevia and different sugars which are low carb in nature.
- Fats like MCT oil, coconut oil, red palm oil and etc.

## Foods which are not allowed

The following classifications of food are not permitted while following the keto diet plan. These foods are high in their carb content and can negatively affect your arrangement:

- Legumes like peas, lentils, and dark beans, and so on.
- Grains like rice, wheat, and corn, and so on.
- Sugar-rich sustenance like maple syrup, agave, and nectar and so on.
- Tubers like yams and potatoes and etc.
- Fruits like oranges, bananas, and apples and etc.
- Sodas, carbonated drinks, sweetened tea or coffee, etc.
- Processed meat and poultry.

## Worse Fats for Keto Diet

Strictly avoid using these oils and fats while being on the Keto diet plan:

- Canola Oil
- Grape-seed Oil
- Corn Oil
- Soybean Oil

- Peanut Oil
- Safflower Oil
- Rapeseed Oil
- Sunflower Oil

## **Hidden Carb Sources and Measures to Avoid Them**

Limiting pasta, cake, and bread are the natural initial steps for lowering down the blood sugar levels of your body. The important thing is that carbs are usually present in foods you generally won't have the slightest idea about. Usually, people having diabetic issues go for 25 to 60 grams of carb per meal. Though, it is advised to consult a doctor to devise the exact amount of carbs your body requires.

- **Milk Alternatives**

    The best alternatives for a dairy intolerant individual are almond milk and soy milk. The important thing to note is to look for sugar quantities in the flavored variants. For instance, a single cup of chocolate soy milk has 23 grams of carbs, while the plain soy milk has only 12 grams of it.

- **Yogurt**

    Yogurt is a well-known source of calcium and is rich in good bacteria known as probiotics. There are a few low-fat, flavored variants having up to 40 grams of carb in every 8 oz. serving. For having a relatively low-carb substitute, I prefer Greek yogurt. The plain, no-fat variant of Greek yogurt has 9 grams of carbs for a similar quantity apart from having more protein.

- **Baked Beans**

    A single cup of baked beans (canned) has a fairly high, i.e., 54 grams of carbs, which can be approximately equal to the entire amount of allowed carbs on a single meal. It is recommended to have a half cup of baked beans as they are rich in protein and dietary fiber too.

- **Tomato Sauce**

    Canned tomato sauces are for sure added with sugar and have around 12 grams of carbs per ½ cup. Always carefully read the nutrition table on the can and note that various brands have high amounts of sodium in them too. In the case of ambiguities, simply spread the sauce on your whole-grain pasta sparingly.

- **Salad Dressing**

    It is important to read the nutrition table before having your salad dressing be it Russian, French, Italian, or Caesar. It is recommended to prepare your own salad dressing by using vinegar and olive oil. If not possible, simply follow the preferred serving size as mentioned on the jars. A smaller amount, i.e., 1-2 tbsp. isn't going to affect your blood sugar levels intensely, but more than 1-2 tbsp. might pose a problem for your keto diet.

- **Orange Chicken**

    A standard serving of orange chickens has a whopping 146 grams of carbs. In case you order an orange chicken, prefer a steamed dish over a battered one!

- **Barbecue Sauce**

    Here too, serving plays an important role, i.e., a single tablespoon will give you around 7 grams of carbs. If you consume around half a cup, you will have around 58 grams of carbs solely from the source.

- **Split Pea Soup**

    Peas are starchy in nature and will give you high amounts of carbs, i.e., 26 grams per cup consumed apart from dietary fiber. There is a high amount of salt in various soups too, so prefer having the ones with a reduced amount of sodium.

- **Protein Bars**

    It is generally considered that higher protein content will automatically mean lower carb content, which is in fact not true at all. Those protein bars which are mostly used by athletes and sportsmen are considerably high both in carbs and proteins. If you need a snack before your work out session, alternatively go for a banana with 1 tbsp. of peanut butter.

- **Sugar-Free Cookies**

    It is a myth that sugar-free means carb-free, that's a ridiculous claim. There are various sugar-free cookies which have the same amount of carbs as their regular sugar added counterparts. Always read the nutrition table carefully before making any choices.

## What is suggested for Drinking?

Water is viewed as the most prescribed and ideal refreshment for keto sweethearts. Notwithstanding water, espresso and tea can likewise be devoured, yet it is to be remembered that you don't need to utilize any sugars, sugar inexplicit. A little amount of milk or cream in espresso or tea is satisfactory, yet not the espresso latte. The periodic utilization of a single glass of wine is additionally permitted.

# 30-Day Meal Plan for Weight Loss & Shopping List

(**Note**: All the recipes below are from the book and specifically chosen for weight loss)

## Meal Plan

### Day 1

**Breakfast:** Coconut Cereal
**Lunch:** Bacon & Jalapeño Soup
**Dinner:** Parmesan Halibut
**Appetizer/Snack:** Deviled Eggs
**Dessert:** Key Lime Pie

### Day 2

**Breakfast:** Strawberry Protein Smoothie
**Lunch:** Chicken Stuffed Avocado
**Dinner:** Green Beans Casserole
**Appetizer/Snack:** Tilapia Strips
**Dessert:** Lemon Curd Tart

### Day 3

**Breakfast:** Cheddar Waffles
**Lunch:** Curried Broccoli
**Dinner:** Beef Taco Soup
**Appetizer/Snack:** Chicken Nuggets
**Dessert:** Cream Cake

### Day 4

**Breakfast:** Fruit & Veggie Smoothie
**Lunch:** Buttered Scallops
**Dinner:** Bacon Wrapped Chicken Breast
**Appetizer/Snack:** Zucchini Sticks
**Dessert:** Ricotta Mousse

### Day 5

**Breakfast:** Creamy Porridge
**Lunch:** Eggplant Curry
**Dinner:** Spicy Roasted Turkey
**Appetizer/Snack:** Bacon Scones
**Dessert:** Blackberry Cobbler

### Day 6

**Breakfast:** Cucumber & Parsley Smoothie
**Lunch:** Pan Fried Squid
**Dinner:** Chocolate Chili
**Appetizer/Snack:** Chicken Popcorn
**Dessert:** Chocolate Panna Cota

## Day 7
**Breakfast:** Chives Scramble
**Lunch:** Tomato & Mozzarella Salad
**Dinner:** Chicken Parmigiana
**Appetizer/Snack:** Cucumber Cups
**Dessert:** Coffee Granita

## Day 8
**Breakfast:** Blackberry Smoothie
**Lunch:** Cauliflower Soup
**Dinner:** Beef Taco Bake
**Appetizer/Snack:** 3 Cheese Crackers
**Dessert:** Matcha Egg Roll Cake

## Day 9
**Breakfast:** Cream Cheese Pancakes
**Lunch:** Stuffed Zucchini
**Dinner:** Coconut Tilapia
**Appetizer/Snack:** Mozzarella Sticks
**Dessert:** Lemon Soufflé

## Day 10
**Breakfast:** Pumpkin Smoothie
**Lunch:** Feta Turkey Burgers
**Dinner:** Shepherd Pie
**Appetizer/Snack:** Cinnamon Cookies
**Dessert:** Cream Fudge

## Day 11
**Breakfast:** Blueberry Bread
**Lunch:** Tomato & Basil Soup
**Dinner:** Cod & Veggies Bake
**Appetizer/Snack:** Bacon Wrapped Asparagus
**Dessert:** Strawberry Sundae

## Day 12
**Breakfast:** Raspberry Smoothie
**Lunch:** Chicken Kabobs
**Dinner:** Lamb Chops with Cream Sauce
**Appetizer/Snack:** Tuna Croquettes
**Dessert:** No-Bake Cheesecake

## Day 13
**Breakfast:** Buttered Crepes
**Lunch:** Braised Cabbage
**Dinner:** Cheesy Pork Cutlets
**Appetizer/Snack:** Walnut Bark
**Dessert:** Key Lime Pie

## Day 14
**Breakfast:** Chocolaty Veggie Smoothie
**Lunch:** Broiled Lamb Chops
**Dinner:** Chicken & Salsa Soup
**Appetizer/Snack:** Avocado Salsa
**Dessert:** Cream Tartlets

### Day 15
**Breakfast:** Spinach Quiche
**Lunch:** Steamed Clams
**Dinner:** Chicken in Creamy Spinach Sauce
**Appetizer/Snack:** Cheesy Tomato Slices
**Dessert:** Mocha Ice Cream

### Day 16
**Breakfast:** Blueberry Smoothie
**Lunch:** Zucchini Pizza
**Dinner:** Pork with Brussels Sprout
**Appetizer/Snack:** Almond Brittles
**Dessert:** Chocolate Pudding

### Day 17
**Breakfast:** Cream Cheese Muffins
**Lunch:** Salad Wraps
**Dinner:** Turkey Casserole
**Appetizer/Snack:** Parmesan Chicken Wings
**Dessert:** Lemon Curd Tart

### Day 18
**Breakfast:** Avocado & Spinach Smoothie
**Lunch:** Creamy Ground Turkey
**Dinner:** Steak with Blueberry Sauce
**Appetizer/Snack:** Broccoli Tots
**Dessert:** Ricotta Mousse

### Day 19
**Breakfast:** Zucchini & Bacon Hash
**Lunch:** Mixed Veggie Combo
**Dinner:** Pork Pinwheel
**Appetizer/Snack:** Mini Salmon Bites
**Dessert:** Matcha Egg Roll Cake

### Day 20
**Breakfast:** Blueberry & Lettuce Smoothie
**Lunch:** Lemony Crab Legs
**Dinner:** Spicy Steak Curry
**Appetizer/Snack:** Cheese Bites
**Dessert:** Mascarpone Brownies

### Day 21
**Breakfast:** Chicken Frittata
**Lunch:** Cauliflower Soup
**Dinner:** Herbed Sardines
**Appetizer/Snack:** Stuffed Tomatoes
**Dessert:** Mocha Ice Cream

### Day 22
**Breakfast:** Chocolate Smoothie
**Lunch:** Grilled Lamb Burgers
**Dinner:** Veggie Loaf
**Appetizer/Snack:** Buffalo Chicken Bites
**Dessert:** Cream Cheese Flan

## Day 23

**Breakfast:** Avocado Cups
**Lunch:** Spinach in Cheese Sauce
**Dinner:** Roasted Whole Chicken
**Appetizer/Snack:** Cauliflower Popcorn
**Dessert:** Chocolate Lava Cake

## Day 24

**Breakfast:** Mixed Berries Smoothie
**Lunch:** Shrimp with Asparagus
**Dinner:** Braised Pork Shanks
**Appetizer/Snack:** Mini Mushroom Pizzas
**Dessert:** Cream Fudge

## Day 25

**Breakfast:** Yogurt Waffles
**Lunch:** Berries & Spinach Salad
**Dinner:** Butter Chicken
**Appetizer/Snack:** Jalapeño Poppers
**Dessert:** Vanilla Crème Soufflé

## Day 26

**Breakfast:** Vanilla Smoothie
**Lunch:** Creamy Brussels Sprout
**Dinner:** Grouper Casserole
**Appetizer/Snack:** Cheese Chips
**Dessert:** Strawberry Sundae

## Day 27

**Breakfast:** Creamy Porridge
**Lunch:** Meatballs in Tomato Gravy
**Dinner:** Zucchini Gratin
**Appetizer/Snack:** Bacon Wrapped Scallops
**Dessert:** Mascarpone Custard

## Day 28

**Breakfast:** Green Veggies Smoothie
**Lunch:** Buttered Lobster Tails
**Dinner:** Beef with Mushroom Gravy
**Appetizer/Snack:** Cheese Balls
**Dessert:** Blackberry Cobbler

## Day 29

**Breakfast:** Seeds Granola
**Lunch:** Green Veggies Soup
**Dinner:** Grilled Leg of Lamb
**Appetizer/Snack:** Cheddar Biscuits
**Dessert:** Vanilla Crème Brûlée

## Day 30

**Breakfast:** Strawberry Smoothie
**Lunch:** Turkey Pizza
**Dinner:** Spinach Pie
**Appetizer/Snack:** Sesame Seeds Crackers
**Dessert:** Coffee Granita

# Shopping List

(**Note**: The lists are listed according to the number of servings in the recipes)

## Poultry

1 (3-pounds) grass-fed whole chicken

3 pounds grass-fed chicken meat

7 pounds grass-fed skinless, boneless chicken breasts

½ pound grass-fed chicken thighs

1 pound grass-fed chicken tenders

3 pounds grass-fed chicken wings

1 pound grass-fed ground chicken

1 (9-pounds) whole turkey

3 pounds ground turkey

126 organic eggs

## Red Meat

3 pounds grass-fed ground beef

2 pounds grass-fed round steak

24 ounces grass-fed flank steaks

1 (4½-pounds) grass-fed boneless leg of lamb

1½ pounds grass-fed lamb chops

8 (4-ounces) grass-fed lamb loin chops

1 pound grass-fed ground lamb

3 pounds pork shoulder

2¼ pounds pork cutlets

1 1/3 pounds pork belly

4 pounds lean ground pork

10 ounces gluten-free pork sausage

1 gluten-free chorizo link

73 bacon slices

16 pepperoni slices

## Fish/Seafood

8 ounces salmon

25 ounces grouper

12 ounces halibut fillets

3 pounds 1 ounce tilapia fillets

24 ounces cod steaks

24 ounces canned white tuna

1 pound shrimp

2 pounds fresh scallops

1 pound squid

1 pound fresh clams

2 (6-ounce) lobster tails

1 pound king crab legs

## Vegetables

1 pumpkin

1 eggplant

18 zucchinis

1 head red cabbage

1 head green cabbage

3 heads broccoli

1 (16-ounces) package frozen chopped broccoli

3 heads cauliflower

2 (12-ounces) packages riced cauliflower

1 red bell pepper

6 green bell peppers

1 pound frozen okra

4 packages fresh spinach

56 ounces packaged frozen spinach

2½ pounds fresh baby spinach

1½ pounds button mushrooms

½ pound fresh cremini mushrooms

4 large Portobello mushrooms

2½ pounds fresh Brussels sprouts

1 pound fresh green beans

1 bunch asparagus

1 (8-ounces) package frozen asparagus spears

5 carrots

3 cucumbers

1 English cucumber

10 celery stalks

22 tomatoes

1 plum tomato

1 (14-ounces) can sugar-free diced tomatoes

1 (28-ounces) can sugar-free plum tomatoes

1 (14½-ounce) can petite diced tomatoes

2 (10-ounces) cans sugar-free diced tomatoes and green chilies

4 pounds cherry tomatoes

22 yellow onions

1 shallot

18 scallions

5 garlic heads

3 knobs fresh ginger

1 head romaine lettuce

3 heads lettuce

26 jalapeño peppers

3 Serrano peppers

1 green chili

1 can chopped green chilies

13 bunches fresh parsley

2 bunches fresh thyme

8 bunches fresh cilantro

3 bunches fresh oregano

3 bunches fresh rosemary

8 bunches fresh basil

2 bunches fresh chives

1 bunch fresh dill

19 lemons

8 limes

## **Fruits**

4 ounces frozen strawberries

6 bags fresh strawberries

4 bags fresh raspberries

5 bags fresh blueberries

3 bags fresh blackberries

9 avocados

## Dairy Products

3 tubs plain Greek yogurt

2 tubs mayonnaise

10 packages cream cheese

2 packages mascarpone cheese

9 containers heavy whipping cream

2 containers whipped cream

14 containers heavy cream

2 containers sour cream

9 packages cheddar cheese

2 packages sharp cheddar cheese

1 package strong cheddar cheese

1 package Muenster cheese

8 packages Parmesan cheese

1 package Parmesan and Romano cheese blend

8 packages mozzarella cheese

1 package part-skim fresh mozzarella cheese

1 package Swiss cheese

1 package pepper jack cheese

1 package Romano cheese

2 packages provolone cheese

4 packages feta cheese

2 packages ricotta cheese

2 package cottage cheese

3 tubs salted butter

6 tubs unsalted butter

8 tubs butter

## Spices & Seasoning

3 bottles salt

1 bottle sea salt

1 bottle coarse salt

1 bottle pumpkin pie spice

1 bottle ground cinnamon

1 bottle ground nutmeg

1 bottle ground ginger

1 bottle ground cloves

1 bottle ground cardamom

1 bottle ground cumin

1 bottle ground coriander

1 bottle ground turmeric

1 bottle garam masala

1 bottle garlic powder

1 bottle red pepper flakes

1 bottle smoked paprika

1 bottle cayenne pepper

1 bottle red chili powder

1 bottle black pepper

1 bottle white pepper

1 bottle curry powder

1 bottle cumin seeds

1 bottle Italian seasoning

1 bottle taco seasoning

1 bottle Cajun seasoning

1 bottle pork seasoning

1 bottle dried onion

1 bottle dried garlic

1 bottle dried oregano

1 bottle dried thyme

1 bottle dried parsley

1 bottle dried dill weed

1 bottle dried rosemary

## **Others**

12 cans unsweetened almond milk

6 cans unsweetened coconut milk

1 tub almond butter

1 tub peanut butter

1 tub natural peanut butter

1 tub unsalted peanut butter

1 jar salsa verde

1 bottle sugar-free ranch dressing

1 bottle Italian dressing

1 bottle hot sauce

2 jars sugar-free BBQ sauce

2 jars sugar-free marinara sauce

3 jars sugar-free tomato sauce

4 jars sugar-free tomato paste

2 bottles olive oil

1 bottle coconut oil

1 bottle MCT oil

Olive oil nonstick cooking spray

1 bottle low-sodium soy sauce

1 bottle Worcestershire sauce

1 bottle balsamic vinegar

3 bottles organic vanilla extract

1 package vanilla bean

3 bags unsweetened coconut flakes

1 bag unsweetened dried coconut

1 bag desiccated coconut

1 bag coconut flour

1 bag almond meal

2 bags almond flour

1 bag superfine blanched almond flour

1 bag coconut flour

1 bag arrowroot powder

1 bag raw sunflower seeds

1 bag flax seeds

1 bag sesame seeds

1 bag golden flax seed meal

1 bag psyllium husk

1 bag psyllium husk powder

2 bottles cacao powder

1 bottle xanthan gum

1 bottle chia seed

1 bag walnuts

1 bag almonds

1 bottle ground mustard

1 bottle mustard

1 bottle organic baking powder

1 bottle baking soda

1 bottle cream of tartar

1 bottle unsweetened whey protein powder

1 bottle unsweetened vanilla whey protein powder

2 bags 70% dark chocolate

1 bottle Dijon mustard

1 bottle poppy seeds

1 package unflavored powdered gelatin

1 bottle instant coffee

1 bottle strong coffee

1 bottle espresso powder

1 bottle matcha powder

2 bags Erythritol

1 bag powdered Erythritol

1 bag Swerve

1 bag powdered Swerve

1 bottle stevia powder

1 bottle liquid stevia

1 bottle monk fruit extract drops

# CHAPTER 1 | SMOOTHIES & BREAKFAST

## Strawberry Smoothie

(**Yields:** 2 servings / **Preparation Time:** 10 minutes)

### Ingredients

- 4 ounces frozen strawberries
- 2 teaspoons Erythritol*
- ½ teaspoon organic vanilla extract
- 1/3 cup heavy whipping cream
- 1¼ cups unsweetened almond milk
- ½ cup ice cubes

### Instructions

1. Place all the ingredients in a high-speed blender and pulse until smooth.
2. Pour the smoothie into serving glasses and serve.

### Nutrition Values (Per Serving)

- Calories: 116
- Net Carbs: 5g
- Carbohydrate: 6.8g
- Fiber: 1.8g
- Protein: 1g
- Fat: 9.6g
- Sugar: 3.5g
- Sodium: 120mg

(**Note: Erythritol*** - Erythritol is a sugar alcohol that is considered safe as a food additive and keto friendly in the United States and throughout much of the world.)

---

## Strawberry Protein Smoothie

(**Yields:** 2 servings / **Preparation Time:** 10 minutes)

### Ingredients

- ½ cup fresh strawberries, hulled and sliced
- 1 scoop unsweetened whey protein powder
- 1 teaspoon chia seed
- 3 tablespoons heavy cream
- 2 teaspoons Erythritol
- ¼ teaspoon organic vanilla extract
- 1½ cups unsweetened almond milk
- ½ cup ice cubes

### Instructions

1. Place all the ingredients in a high-speed blender and pulse until smooth.
2. Pour the smoothie into serving glasses and serve.

### Nutrition Values (Per Serving)

- Calories: 178
- Net Carbs: 3.6g
- Carbohydrate: 7.1g
- Fiber: 3.5g
- Protein: 13g
- Fat: 11.7g
- Sugar: 2.5g
- Sodium: 170mg

---

## Blackberry Smoothie

**(Yields:** 2 servings / **Preparation Time:** 10 minutes)

### Ingredients

- 2 ounces fresh blackberries
- 2 ounces cream cheese, softened
- ¼ cup heavy cream
- 3-5 drops liquid stevia
- ½ teaspoon organic vanilla extract
- ¾ cup unsweetened almond milk
- ½ cup ice cubes

### Instructions

1. Add all the ingredients in a high-speed blender and pulse until smooth.
2. Pour the smoothie into serving glasses and serve.

### Nutrition Values (Per Serving)

- Calories: 181
- Net Carbs: 2.9g
- Carbohydrate: 4.8g
- Fiber: 1.9g
- Protein: 3.2g
- Fat: 16.9g
- Sugar: 1.6g
- Sodium: 159mg

(**Tip:** To increase the protein content, you can add one scoop of unsweetened protein powder.)

---

## Raspberry Smoothie

**(Yields:** 2 servings / **Preparation Time:** 10 minutes)

### Ingredients

- ½ cup fresh raspberries
- ¼ cup heavy whipping cream
- 1 tablespoon cream cheese
- 2 tablespoons Erythritol
- ½ teaspoon organic vanilla extract
- Pinch of salt
- 1¼ cups unsweetened almond milk
- ½ cup ice cubes

### Instructions

1. Place all the ingredients in a high-speed blender and pulse until smooth.
2. Pour the smoothie into serving glasses and serve.

### Nutrition Values (Per Serving)

- Calories: 113
- Net Carbs: 3g
- Carbohydrate: 5.6g
- Fiber: 2.6g
- Protein: 1.7g
- Fat: 9.7g
- Sugar: 1.5g
- Sodium: 211mg

---

## Blueberry Smoothie

**(Yields:** 2 servings / **Preparation Time:** 10 minutes)

### Ingredients

- ½ cup fresh blueberries
- 2 teaspoons MCT oil
- ½ teaspoon organic vanilla extract
- 2-4 drops liquid stevia
- 1¾ cups unsweetened almond milk
- ½ cup ice cubes

### Instructions

1. Add all the ingredients in a high-speed blender and pulse until smooth.
2. Pour the smoothie into serving glasses and serve.

### Nutrition Values (Per Serving)

- Calories: 92
- Net Carbs: 5.1g
- Carbohydrate: 7g
- Fiber: 1.9g
- Protein: 1.2g
- Fat: 7.9g
- Sugar: 3.7g
- Sodium: 158mg

(**Tip:** For a thicker smoothie, you can add 2-3 tablespoons of yogurt.)

# Blueberry & Lettuce Smoothie

**(Yields:** 2 servings / **Preparation Time:** 10 minutes)

## Ingredients

- 1/3 cup fresh blueberries
- 1¼ cups romaine lettuce, chopped
- 4-6 drops liquid stevia
- 1½ cups unsweetened almond milk
- ½ cup ice cubes

## Instructions

1. Place all the ingredients in a high-speed blender and pulse until smooth.
2. Pour the smoothie into serving glasses and serve.

## Nutrition Values (Per Serving)

- Calories: 49
- Net Carbs: 4.2g
- Carbohydrate: 6g
- Fiber: 1.8g
- Protein: 1.1g
- Fat: 2.8g
- Sugar: 2.7g
- Sodium: 139mg

---

# Mixed Berries Smoothie

**(Yields:** 2 servings / **Preparation Time:** 10 minutes)

## Ingredients

- ¼ cup fresh strawberries
- ¼ cup fresh blackberries
- ¼ cup fresh raspberries
- 1 tablespoon unsweetened coconut, shredded
- 1-2 packets stevia powder
- 1/3 cup cottage cheese
- 1½ cups unsweetened almond milk

## Instructions

1. Add all the ingredients in a high-speed blender and pulse until smooth.
2. Pour the smoothie into serving glasses and serve.

## Nutrition Values (Per Serving)

- Calories: 94
- Net Carbs: 4.9g
- Carbohydrate: 8.2g
- Fiber: 3.3g
- Protein: 6.6g
- Fat: 4.4g
- Sugar: 2.7g
- Sodium: 289mg

(**Tip:** Make sure to wash the berries thoroughly.)

# Vanilla Smoothie

**(Yields:** 2 servings / **Preparation Time:** 5 minutes)

## Ingredients

- ½ cup unsweetened vanilla whey protein powder
- 4 tablespoons almond butter
- 2 teaspoons organic vanilla extract
- 6-8 drops liquid stevia
- 2 cups unsweetened almond milk
- ½ cup ice cubes

## Instructions

1. Place all the ingredients in a high-speed blender and pulse until smooth.
2. Pour the smoothie into serving glasses and serve.

## Nutrition Values (Per Serving)

- Calories: 369
- Net Carbs: 6g
- Carbohydrate: 10g
- Fiber: 4g
- Protein: 34.7g
- Fat: 22.7g
- Sugar: 2.5g
- Sodium: 225mg

(**Tip:** Be sure to use high quality and unsweetened protein powder.)

---

# Chocolate Smoothie

**(Yields:** 3 servings / **Preparation Time:** 10 minutes)

## Ingredients

- 3 tablespoons cacao powder
- 4 tablespoons powdered Erythritol
- Pinch of salt
- 1 cup heavy cream
- ¼ cup creamy peanut butter
- 1½ cups unsweetened almond milk

## Instructions

1. Place all the ingredients in a high-speed blender and pulse until smooth.
2. Pour the smoothie into serving glasses and serve.

## Nutrition Values (Per Serving)

- Calories: 297
- Net Carbs: 5.3g
- Carbohydrate: 8.7g
- Fiber: 3.4g
- Protein: 7.7g
- Fat: 28.4g
- Sugar: 2.1g
- Sodium: 282mg

(**Tip:** For an extra boost, you can supplement with unsweetened protein powder.)

# Pumpkin Smoothie

**(Yields:** 2 servings / **Preparation Time:** 10 minutes)

## Ingredients

- ½ cup homemade pumpkin puree
- 1 scoop unsweetened whey protein powder
- ¼ teaspoon pumpkin pie spice
- 1½ tablespoons Erythritol
- ½ tablespoon MCT oil
- ½ cup heavy whipping cream
- 1 cup unsweetened almond milk
- ½ cup ice cubes

## Instructions

1. Add all the ingredients in a high-speed blender and pulse until smooth.
2. Pour the smoothie into serving glasses and serve.

## Nutrition Values (Per Serving)

- Calories: 223
- Net Carbs: 5.2g
- Carbohydrate: 7.7g
- Fiber: 2.5g
- Protein: 12.8g
- Fat: 17.2g
- Sugar: 2.7g
- Sodium: 129mg

**(Tip:** MCT oil can be replaced with coconut oil.)

---

# Cucumber & Parsley Smoothie

**(Yields:** 2 servings / **Preparation Time:** 10 minutes)

## Ingredients

- 1½ cups cucumber, peeled and chopped
- 1 cup fresh parsley leaves
- 1 (1-inch) piece fresh ginger, peeled and chopped
- 2 tablespoons fresh lemon juice
- 4-6 drops liquid stevia
- 1½ cups chilled water

## Instructions

1. Place all the ingredients in a high-speed blender and pulse until smooth.
2. Pour the smoothie into serving glasses and serve.

## Nutrition Values (Per Serving)

- Calories: 25
- Net Carbs: 3.7g

- Carbohydrate: 5.1g
- Fiber: 1.4g
- Protein: 1.4g
- Fat: 0.4g
- Sugar: 1.6g
- Sodium: 19mg

## **Avocado & Spinach Smoothie**

**(Yields:** 2 servings / **Preparation Time:** 10 minutes)

### Ingredients

- ½ large avocado, peeled, pitted and roughly chopped
- 2 cups fresh spinach
- 1 tablespoon MCT oil
- 1 teaspoon organic vanilla extract
- 6-8 drops liquid stevia
- 1½ cups unsweetened almond milk
- ½ cup ice cubes

### Instructions

1. Place all the ingredients in a high-speed blender and pulse until smooth.
2. Pour the smoothie into serving glasses and serve.

### Nutrition Values (Per Serving)

- Calories: 195
- Net Carbs: 2.4g
- Carbohydrate: 7.2g
- Fiber: 4.8g
- Protein: 2.6g
- Fat: 19.6g
- Sugar: 0.7g
- Sodium: 162mg

## **Green Veggies Smoothie**

**(Yields:** 2 servings / **Preparation Time:** 10 minutes)

### Ingredients

- 1 cup fresh spinach
- ¼ cup broccoli florets, chopped
- ¼ cup green cabbage, chopped
- ½ of small green bell pepper, seeded and chopped
- 8-10 drops liquid stevia
- 1½ cups chilled water

### Instructions

1. Place all the ingredients in a high-speed blender and pulse until smooth.
2. Pour the smoothie into serving glasses and serve.

### Nutrition Values (Per Serving)

- Calories: 19
- Net Carbs: 2.8g
- Carbohydrate: 4.1g
- Fiber: 1.3g
- Protein: 1.2g
- Fat: 0.2g
- Sugar: 2g
- Sodium: 18mg

(**Tip:** Make sure to use fresh vegetables for a better taste.)

---

## Fruit & Veggies Smoothie

(**Yields:** 2 servings / **Preparation Time:** 10 minutes)

### Ingredients

- ¼ cup fresh raspberries
- ¼ cup fresh strawberries, hulled
- ½ of red bell pepper, seeded and chopped
- ¼ cup red cabbage, chopped
- 6-8 drops liquid stevia
- 1½ cups water
- ½ cup ice cubes

### Instructions

1. Place all the ingredients in a high-speed blender and pulse until smooth.
2. Pour the smoothie into serving glasses and serve.

### Nutrition Values (Per Serving)

- Calories: 22
- Net Carbs: 3g
- Carbohydrate: 5.1g
- Fiber: 2.1g
- Protein: 0.7g
- Fat: 5.1g
- Sugar: 2.5g
- Sodium: 3mg

---

## Chocolaty Veggie Smoothie

(**Yields:** 2 servings / **Preparation Time:** 10 minutes)

### Ingredients

- 1 cup fresh spinach, chopped
- ½ cup zucchini, peeled and roughly chopped
- 3 tablespoons cacao powder
- 2 tablespoons unsalted peanut butter
- 2 tablespoons Erythritol
- 2 cups chilled water

## Instructions

1. Add all the ingredients in a high-speed blender and pulse until smooth.
2. Pour the smoothie into serving glasses and serve.

## Nutrition Values (Per Serving)

- Calories: 121
- Net Carbs: 4.6g
- Carbohydrate: 8.4g
- Fiber: 3.8g
- Protein: 6.3g
- Fat: 9.7g
- Sugar: 2.1g
- Sodium: 88mg

---

# Seeds Granola

**(Yields:** 15 servings / **Prep Time:** 15 minutes / **Cooking Time:** 20 minutes)

## Ingredients

- 3 cups unsweetened coconut flakes
- 1 cup walnuts, chopped
- ½ cup flaxseeds
- 2/3 cup pumpkin seeds
- 2/3 cup sunflower seeds
- ¼ cup butter, melted
- 1 teaspoon ground ginger
- 1 teaspoon ground cinnamon
- 1/8 teaspoon ground cloves
- 1/8 teaspoon ground cardamom
- Pinch of salt

## Instructions

1. Preheat the oven to 350 degrees F. Lightly grease a large rimmed baking sheet.
2. In a bowl, add the coconut flakes, walnuts, flaxseeds, pumpkin seeds, sunflower seeds, butter, spices, and salt and toss to coat well.
3. Transfer mixture onto the prepared baking sheet and spread in an even layer.
4. Bake for about 20 minutes, stirring after every 3-4 minutes.
5. Remove the baking sheet of granola from oven and let it cool completely before serving.
6. Break the granola into desired size chunks and serve with your favorite non-dairy milk.

## Nutrition Values (Per Serving)

- Calories: 200
- Net Carbs: 3.1g
- Carbohydrate: 6.8g
- Fiber: 3.7g
- Protein: 5.5g
- Fat: 17.8g
- Sugar: 0.3g
- Sodium: 36mg

**(Tip:** You can preserve this granola into an airtight container for up to 2 weeks.)

# Coconut Cereal

(**Yields:** 16 servings / **Prep Time:** 10 minutes / **Cooking Time:** 25 minutes)

## Ingredients

- 1 tablespoon ground cinnamon
- 1 teaspoon ground nutmeg
- 1 tablespoon organic vanilla extract
- ½ teaspoon stevia powder
- ½ cup water
- 1 pound unsweetened coconut flakes

## Instructions

1. Preheat the oven to 300 degrees F. Line 2-3 cookie sheets with parchment paper.
2. Place all the ingredients in a large bowl and beat until well combined.
3. Transfer coconut flakes evenly onto the prepared cookie sheets and spread into an even layer.
4. Bake for about 15 minutes.
5. Remove all the cookie sheets from oven and stir the flakes.
6. Bake for about 5-10 more minutes.
7. Remove all the cookie sheets from oven and set aside to cool completely.
8. Serve with your favorite non-dairy milk.

## Nutrition Values (Per Serving)

- Calories: 136
- Net Carbs: 4.1g
- Carbohydrate: 8.1g
- Fiber: 4g
- Protein: 1.9g
- Fat: 11.4g
- Sugar: 0.2g
- Sodium: 0mg

(**Tip:** The topping of fresh berries will enhance the flavor of this coconut cereal.)

---

# Creamy Porridge

(**Yields:** 3 servings / **Prep Time:** 15 minutes / **Cooking Time:** 10 minutes)

## Ingredients

- 1½ cups water
- 1/3 cup almond flour
- 2 tablespoons flax seed meal
- Pinch of salt
- 2 organic eggs, beaten
- 2 tablespoons heavy cream
- 2 tablespoons Erythritol
- 4 teaspoons unsalted butter
- 3 tablespoons fresh blueberries

## Instructions

1. In a pan, add the water, almond flour, flax meal, and salt over medium-high heat and bring to a boil, stirring continuously.
2. Now, set the heat to medium and cook for about 2-3 minutes, beating continuously.
3. Remove from heat and slowly, add the beaten eggs, beating continuously.
4. Return the pan over medium heat and cook for about 2-3 minutes or until the mixture becomes thick.
5. Remove from the heat and beat for at least 30 seconds.
6. Add the heavy cream, Erythritol, and butter and beat until well combined.
7. Top with the blueberries and serve immediately.

## Nutrition Values (Per Serving)

- Calories: 221
- Net Carbs: 3.3g
- Carbohydrate: 6.2g
- Fiber: 2.9g
- Protein: 7.7g
- Fat: 19.6g
- Sugar: 1.6g
- Sodium: 159mg

---

# Pumpkin Porridge

**(Yields:** 4 servings / **Prep Time:** 15 minutes / **Cooking Time:** 4 minutes)

## Ingredients

- ¼ cup homemade pumpkin puree
- 1/3 cup almond flour
- 2 tablespoons coconut flour
- 2 teaspoons ground flax seed
- 2 tablespoons Erythritol
- ½ teaspoon pumpkin pie spice
- ½ teaspoon ground cinnamon
- ½ teaspoon salt
- ¼ cup half-and-half
- ¾ cup water
- ¼ cup fresh strawberries, hulled and sliced

## Instructions

1. Add all the ingredients except strawberry slices into a small pan and with a wire whisk, beat until well combined.
2. Now, place the pan over medium heat and cook for about 3-4 minutes or until heated through, stirring continuously.
3. Remove the pan of porridge from heat and let it cool for about 5 minutes.
4. Transfer the porridge evenly into serving bowls.
5. Top with strawberry slices and serve.

### Nutrition Values (Per Serving)

- Calories: 113
- Net Carbs: 4.2g
- Carbohydrate: 8g
- Fiber: 3.8g
- Protein: 3.7g
- Fat: 7.6g
- Sugar: 1g
- Sodium: 303mg

---

## Cheddar Waffles

**(Yields:** 8 servings / **Prep Time:** 15 minutes / **Total Cooking Time:** 48 minutes)

### Ingredients

- 1 cup golden flax seed meal
- 1 cup almond flour
- ¼ cup unflavored whey protein powder
- 2 teaspoons baking powder
- Salt and ground black pepper, as required
- 1½ cups cheddar cheese, shredded
- ¾ cup unsweetened almond milk
- ¼ cup unsalted butter, melted
- 4 large organic eggs, beaten
- 2 tablespoons butter, softened

### Instructions

1. Preheat waffle iron and grease it.
2. In a large bowl, mix well flax seed meal, flour, protein powder, baking powder, salt and black pepper.
3. Stir in the cheddar cheese.
4. In another bowl, add the almond milk, melted butter, and eggs and beat until well combined.
5. Add egg mixture into the bowl of flour mixture and mix until well combined.
6. Place desired amount of mixture into the preheated waffle iron.
7. Cook for about 4-6 minutes or until golden brown.
8. Repeat with the remaining mixture.
9. Serve warm with the topping of softened butter.

### Nutrition Values (Per Serving)

- Calories: 394
- Net Carbs: 4g
- Carbohydrate: 10.3g
- Fiber: 6.3g
- Protein: 19.1g
- Fat: 31.1g
- Sugar: 0.3g
- Sodium: 216mg

# Cream Cheese Pancakes

**(Yields:** 4 servings / **Prep Time:** 10 minutes / **Total Cooking Time:** 12 minutes**)**

## Ingredients

- 2 organic eggs
- 2 ounces cream cheese, softened
- ½ teaspoon ground cinnamon
- 1 packet stevia
- Olive oil nonstick cooking spray

## Instructions

1. Place all the ingredients in a blender and pulse until smooth.
2. Transfer the mixture into a bowl and set aside for about 2-3 minutes.
3. Grease a large nonstick skillet with cooking spray and heat over medium heat.
4. Add ¼ of the mixture and tilt the pan to spread it in an even layer.
5. Cook for about 2 minutes or until golden brown.
6. Flip the side and cook for about 1 more minute.
7. Repeat with the remaining mixture.
8. Serve warm.

## Nutrition Values (Per Serving)

- Calories: 82
- Net Carbs: 0.8g
- Carbohydrate: 0.8g
- Fiber: 0g
- Protein: 3.8g
- Fat: 73g
- Sugar: 0g
- Sodium: 160mg

(**Tip:** Grease the bottom of cooking pan to avoid the sticking of pancakes.)

---

# Spinach Pancakes

**(Yields:** 8 servings / **Prep Time:** 15 minutes / **Total Cooking Time:** 56 minutes**)**

## Ingredients

- 2 organic eggs
- 1 cup almond flour
- ½ teaspoon organic baking powder
- ¼ cup water
- ½ cup feta cheese, crumbled
- 1 cup fresh spinach, chopped
- 2 scallions, chopped
- 1 garlic clove, chopped
- ¼ teaspoon ground nutmeg
- Salt and ground black pepper, as required
- 2 tablespoons unsalted butter

## Instructions

1. Crack the eggs in a bowl and beat until frothy.
2. Add the almond flour, baking powder, and water and beat until smooth.
3. Add the feta cheese, spinach, scallions, garlic, nutmeg, salt, and black pepper and stir to combine.
4. In a large nonstick frying pan, melt ½ tablespoon of butter over medium heat.
5. Add desired amount of the mixture and tilt the pan to spread it in an even layer.
6. Cook for 3-4 minutes or until golden brown.
7. Flip the side and cook for about 2-3 more minutes.
8. Repeat with the remaining butter and spinach mixture.
9. Serve warm.

## Nutrition Values (Per Serving)

- Calories: 179
- Net Carbs: 2.6g
- Carbohydrate: 4.3g
- Fiber: 1.7g
- Protein: 6g
- Fat: 15.6g
- Sugar: 0.6g
- Sodium: 317mg

---

# Cheese Crepes

**(Yields:** 10 servings / **Prep Time:** 20 minutes / **Total Cooking Time:** 20 minutes**)**

## Ingredients

- 6 ounces cream cheese, softened
- 1/3 cup Parmesan cheese, grated
- 6 large organic eggs
- 1 teaspoon Erythritol
- 1½ tablespoons coconut flour
- 1/8 teaspoon xanthan gum
- 2 tablespoons unsalted butter
- 2½ cups fresh strawberries, hulled and sliced

## Instructions

1. In a blender, add the cream cheese, Parmesan cheese, eggs, and Erythritol and pulse on low speed until well combined.
2. While the motor is running, place the coconut flour, and xanthan gum and pulse until a thick mixture is formed.
3. Now, pulse on medium speed for about 5-10 seconds.
4. Transfer the mixture into a bowl and set aside for at least 5 minutes.
5. In a heavy-bottomed frying pan, melt the butter over medium-low heat.
6. Add ¼ cup of mixture and tilt the pan to spread into a thin layer.
7. Cook for about 1½ minutes or until the edges become brown.

8. Carefully, flip the crepe and cook for about 15-20 more seconds.
9. Repeat with the remaining mixture.
10. Serve warm with the filling of strawberry slices.

## Nutrition Values (Per Serving)

- Calories: 171
- Net Carbs: 3.6g
- Carbohydrate: 4.8g
- Fiber: 1.2g
- Protein: 8.7g
- Fat: 13.6g
- Sugar: 2g
- Sodium: 313mg

---

# Buttered Crepes

**(Yields:** 8 servings / **Prep Time:** 15 minutes / **Cooking Time:** 15 minutes)

## Ingredients

**For Crepes:**

- ½ cup unsweetened almond milk
- 4 tablespoons butter, melted
- 6 medium organic eggs
- 3 tablespoons coconut flour
- 3 teaspoons arrowroot powder
- ¼ teaspoon salt
- ½ teaspoon organic vanilla extract
- 4 teaspoons unsalted butter

**For Filling:**

- 6 tablespoons unsweetened coconut milk
- 4 tablespoons unsalted butter
- 1 teaspoon cacao powder
- Pinch of salt

## Instructions

1. For crepes: in a bowl, add the almond milk, melted butter, eggs, flour, arrowroot powder, salt, and vanilla extract and beat until smooth.
2. Set the mixture aside for about 5 minutes.
3. In a cast iron skillet, melt ½ teaspoon of butter over medium heat.
4. Add ¼ cup of mixture and tilt the pan to spread into a thin layer.
5. Cook for 1 minute or until the edges become brown.
6. Carefully, flip the crepe and cook for about 30 more seconds.
7. Repeat with the remaining mixture.
8. Meanwhile: for the filling: in a bowl, add the coconut milk, butter, cacao powder, and salt and beat until smooth and creamy.
9. Serve the crepes with the filling of butter mixture.

### Nutrition Values (Per Serving)

- Calories: 207
- Net Carbs: 2.5g
- Carbohydrate: 4g
- Fiber: 1.5g
- Protein: 5g
- Fat: 3.1g
- Sugar: 0.7g
- Sodium: 244mg

**(Tip:** Remember to beat the crepes mixture for about 10 seconds before pouring into the skillet.)

---

## Cream Cheese Muffins

**(Yields:** 5 servings / **Prep Time:** 15 minutes / **Cooking Time:** 20 minutes)

### Ingredients

- 2 (8-ounces) packages cream cheese
- ½ cup Erythritol
- 2 organic eggs
- ½ teaspoon organic vanilla extract
- 1 teaspoon ground cinnamon

### Instructions

1. Preheat the oven to 350 degrees F. Grease 10 cups of a muffin tin.
2. In a bowl, add the cream cheese, Erythritol, eggs, and vanilla extract and beat until smooth.
3. Transfer mixture evenly into the prepared muffin cups and then, sprinkle each with cinnamon.
4. Bake for about 20 minutes or until a wooden skewer inserted in the center comes out clean.
5. Remove the muffin tin from oven and place onto a wire rack to cool for about 10 minutes.
6. Carefully invert the muffins onto a wire rack to cool completely.
7. Serve.

### Nutrition Values (Per Serving)

- Calories: 344
- Net Carbs: 2.8g
- Carbohydrate: 3g
- Fiber: 0.2g
- Protein: 9.1g
- Fat: 33.4g
- Sugar: 04g
- Sodium: 293mg

**(Tip:** You can use a small ice cream scooper to transfer the mixture into muffin cups to avoid the mess.)

# Beef Muffins

**(Yields:** 6 servings / **Prep Time:** 20 minutes / **Cooking Time:** 20 minutes)

## Ingredients

- 1-pound grass-fed ground beef
- ¾ cup sharp cheddar cheese, shredded and divided
- 1/3 cup jalapeño peppers, chopped and divided
- 2 organic eggs
- 1 tablespoon liquid smoke
- 1 teaspoon garlic powder
- 1 teaspoon onion powder
- Salt and ground black pepper, as required

## Instructions

1. Preheat the oven to 350 degrees F. Grease 12 cups of a muffin tin.
2. In a large bowl, mix well beef, ½ cup of cheddar cheese, ¼ cup of jalapeño peppers, eggs, liquid smoke, garlic powder, onion powder, salt, and black pepper.
3. Place mixture evenly into the prepared muffin cups and top each with the remaining jalapeño peppers and cheddar cheese.
4. Bake for 20 minutes or until the top of muffins becomes golden brown.
5. Remove the muffin tin from oven and place onto a wire rack to cool for about 10 minutes.
6. Carefully invert the muffins onto a platter and serve warm.

## Nutrition Values (Per Serving)

- Calories: 223
- Net Carbs: 1g
- Carbohydrate: 1.2g
- Fiber: 0.2g
- Protein: 28.5g
- Fat: 10.9g
- Sugar: 0.6g
- Sodium: 282mg

---

# Blueberry Bread

**(Yields:** 8 servings / **Prep Time:** 15 minutes / **Cooking Time:** 45 minutes)

## Ingredients

- ½ cup almond flour
- 2 teaspoons organic baking powder
- ½ teaspoon salt
- 5 organic eggs
- ½ cup unsweetened almond milk
- ½ cup almond butter, melted
- ½ cup unsalted butter, melted
- ½ cup fresh blueberries

### Instructions

1. Preheat the oven to 350 degrees F. Line a loaf pan with parchment paper.
2. In a bowl, mix well flour, baking powder, and salt.
3. Add the eggs and almond milk in a second bowl and beat well.
4. In a third bowl, mix together the almond butter and butter.
5. Now, add the flour mixture and mix until well combined.
6. Add the egg mixture and mix until well combined.
7. Gently, fold in the blueberries.
8. Place mixture evenly into the prepared bread loaf pan and with your hands, press to smooth the top surface.
9. Bake for 45 minutes or until a wooden skewer inserted in the center comes out clean.
10. Remove the loaf pan from oven and place onto a wire rack to cool for about 10 minutes.
11. Carefully, invert the bread onto a wire rack to cool completely before slicing.
12. With a sharp knife, cut the bread loaf into 8 equal-sized slices and serve.

### Nutrition Values (Per Serving)

- Calories: 196
- Net Carbs: 2.7g
- Carbohydrate: 3.9g
- Fiber: 1.2g
- Protein: 5.4g
- Fat: 12.8g
- Sugar: 1.4g
- Sodium: 280mg

---

## Cheddar Bread

**(Yields:** 16 servings / **Prep Time:** 15 minutes / **Cooking Time:** 55 minutes)

### Ingredients

- 1 cup blanched almond flour
- ½ cup coconut flour
- ¾ teaspoon organic baking powder
- 12 ounces sharp cheddar cheese, shredded
- 3 large organic eggs
- 3 tablespoons MCT oil
- 1 tablespoon savory seasoning*
- ½ teaspoon onion powder
- ½ teaspoon garlic powder
- ½ teaspoon salt

### Instructions

1. Preheat the oven to 375 degrees F. Line a bread loaf pan with parchment paper.
2. In a food processor, put all the ingredients and pulse until well combined.
3. Place mixture evenly into the prepared bread loaf pan and with your hands, press to smooth the top surface.

4. Bake for 52-55 minutes or until a wooden skewer inserted in the center comes out clean.
5. Remove the loaf pan from oven and place onto a wire rack to cool for about 10-15 minutes.
6. Carefully, invert the bread onto wire rack.
7. With a sharp knife, cut the bread loaf into 16 equal-sized slices and serve warm.

## **Nutrition Values (Per Serving)**

- Calories: 176
- Net Carbs: 2.4g
- Carbohydrate: 4.8g
- Fiber: 2.4g
- Protein: 8.5g
- Fat: 14.3g
- Sugar: 0.2g
- Sodium: 222mg

**(Note: Savory seasonings\*** - Savory is an herb used in cooking. Savory seasonings are any herbs with a non-sweet flavor profile, such as parsley, sage, rosemary, thyme or marjoram**.)**

# **Bacon Omelet**

(**Yields:** 1 serving / **Prep Time:** 15 minutes / **Cooking Time:** 14 minutes)

## **Ingredients**

- 1 bacon slice
- ½ tablespoon butter
- 2 large organic eggs
- ½ tablespoon fresh chives, minced
- Ground black pepper, as required
- 1 ounce cheddar cheese, shredded

## **Instructions**

1. Heat a nonstick small skillet over medium-high heat and cook the bacon slice for about 8-10 minutes, stirring frequently.
2. With a slotted spoon, transfer the bacon onto a paper towel-lined plate to drain.
3. Then, chop the bacon slice.
4. Remove the bacon grease from frying pan and then, wipe it using a paper towel.
5. In a bowl, add the eggs, chives, and black pepper and beat until well combined.
6. In the same frying pan, melt the butter over medium-low heat.
7. Add the egg mixture and cook for about 2 minutes.
8. Carefully, flip the side of omelet and top with chopped bacon.
9. Cook for about 1-2 minutes or until desired doneness of eggs.
10. Remove from heat and immediately, add cheese in the center of omelet.
11. Fold the edges of omelet over cheese.
12. Serve immediately.

## Nutrition Values (Per Serving)

- Calories: 466
- Net Carbs: 1.6g
- Carbohydrate: 1.7g
- Fiber: 0.1g
- Protein: 30.5g
- Fat: 37.2g
- Sugar: 1g
- Sodium: 1000mg

(**Tip:** To have the best omelet, make sure to use a round sauté pan with slope sides.)

---

# Chives Scramble

(**Yields:** 6 servings / **Prep Time:** 15 minutes / **Cooking Time:** 8 minutes)

## Ingredients

- 2 tablespoons olive oil
- 1 jalapeño pepper, chopped
- 1 small yellow onion, chopped
- 12 large organic eggs, beaten lightly
- Salt and ground black pepper, as required
- 3 tablespoons fresh chives, finely chopped
- 4 ounces cheddar cheese, shredded

## Instructions

1. Heat the oil in a large skillet over medium heat and sauté the jalapeño pepper and onion for about 4-5 minutes.
2. Add the eggs, salt, and black pepper and cook for about 3 minutes, stirring continuously.
3. Remove the skillet from heat and immediately, stir in the chives and cheese.
4. Serve.

## Nutrition Values (Per Serving)

- Calories: 265
- Net Carbs: 1.9g
- Carbohydrate: 2.3g
- Fiber: 0.4g
- Protein: 17.5g
- Fat: 20.9g
- Sugar: 1.5g
- Sodium: 285mg

(**Tip:** Crack the eggs into a bowl and with a whisk, break apart the yolks before beating them. Cracking the eggs directly into pan will result in a not-soft scramble.)

# Chicken Frittata

**(Yields:** 4 servings / **Prep Time:** 15 minutes / **Cooking Time:** 12 minutes)

## Ingredients

- 1/3 cup Parmesan cheese, grated
- 6 organic eggs, beaten lightly
- Salt and ground black pepper, as required
- 1 teaspoon unsalted butter
- ½ cup grass-fed cooked chicken, chopped
- ½ cup boiled asparagus, chopped
- 1 tablespoon fresh parsley, chopped

## Instructions

1. Preheat the broiler of oven.
2. In a bowl, mix together the cheese, eggs, salt, and black pepper.
3. Melt the butter in a large ovenproof skillet over medium-high heat and cook the chicken and asparagus for about 2-3 minutes.
4. Stir in the egg mixture and cook for about 4-5 minutes.
5. Remove from the heat and then, sprinkle with parsley.
6. Now, transfer the skillet under broiler and broil for about 3-4 minutes or until slightly puffed.
7. Cut into desired size wedges and serve immediately.

## Nutrition Values (Per Serving)

- Calories: 157
- Net Carbs: 0.8g
- Carbohydrate: 1.2g
- Fiber: 0.4g
- Protein: 16.5g
- Fat: 9.7g
- Sugar: 0.8g
- Sodium: 207mg

---

# Spinach Quiche

**(Yields:** 6 servings / **Prep Time:** 15 minutes / **Cooking Time:** 38 minutes)

## Ingredients

- 1 tablespoon butter
- 1 yellow onion, chopped
- 1 (10-ounces) package frozen spinach, thawed
- 5 organic eggs, beaten
- 3 cups Muenster cheese, shredded
- 1/8 teaspoon red pepper flakes, crushed
- Salt and ground black pepper, as required

## Instructions

1. Preheat the oven to 350 degrees F. Lightly grease a 9-inch pie dish.

2. In a large skillet, melt butter over medium heat and sauté the onion for about 4-5 minutes.
3. Add the spinach and stir to combine.
4. Increase the heat to medium-high and cook for about 2-3 minutes or until all the liquid is absorbed.
5. Remove the skillet of spinach mixture from heat and set aside to cool slightly.
6. Meanwhile, in a large bowl, add the remaining ingredients and mix until well combined.
7. Add the spinach mixture and stir to mix well.
8. Transfer mixture into the prepared pie dish.
9. Bake for about 30 minutes.
10. Remove from oven and set aside to cool for about 10 minutes before serving.
11. Cut into 6 equal-sized wedges and serve.

## Nutrition Values (Per Serving)

- Calories: 296
- Net Carbs: 3g
- Carbohydrate: 4.4g
- Fiber: 1.4g
- Protein: 19.4g
- Fat: 22.7g
- Sugar: 1.9g
- Sodium: 485mg

**(Tip:** Make sure that the baking rack is in the middle of oven.)

---

# Zucchini & Bacon Hash

**(Yields:** 1 serving / **Prep Time:** 15 minutes / **Cooking Time:** 25 minutes)

## Ingredients

- 2 tablespoons butter, divided
- 1 garlic clove, finely chopped
- 2 bacon slices, chopped
- 1 medium zucchini, cut into medium pieces
- 1 tablespoon fresh parsley, chopped
- 1 large organic egg
- Salt, as required

## Instructions

1. In a skillet, melt one tablespoon of butter over medium heat and sauté the garlic for about one minute.
2. Add the bacon slices and cook for about 7-8 minutes or until lightly browned, stirring frequently.
3. Add the zucchini and cook for about 10-15 minutes, stirring occasionally.
4. Meanwhile, in a large nonstick frying pan, melt the remaining butter over medium heat.

5. Carefully, crack the egg into frying pan and cook for about 2-2½ minutes, gently tilting the pan occasionally.
6. In the skillet of zucchini, stir in the salt and remove from heat.
7. Transfer the zucchini hash onto a serving plate and top with the egg.
8. Sprinkle the egg with a little salt.
9. Garnish with fresh parsley and serve.

## Nutrition Values (Per Serving)

- Calories: 614
- Net Carbs: 4.9g
- Carbohydrate: 6.4g
- Fiber: 1.5g
- Protein: 29.7g
- Fat: 52.5g
- Sugar: 2.5g
- Sodium: 1500mg

# Avocado Cups

(**Yields:** 4 servings / **Prep Time:** 15 minutes / **Cooking Time:** 15 minutes)

## Ingredients

- 2 ripe avocados, halved lengthwise and pitted
- ½ teaspoon garlic powder
- 4 medium organic eggs
- Salt and ground black pepper, as required
- 2 tablespoons Parmesan cheese, shredded
- 1 teaspoon fresh chives, minced

## Instructions

1. Preheat the oven to 350 degrees F. Line a baking sheet with a piece of foil.
2. Carefully, scoop out 1-2 tablespoons of flesh from the center of each avocado half.
3. Arrange avocado halves onto the prepared baking sheet, cut side up.
4. Sprinkle each avocado half evenly with garlic powder.
5. Carefully, crack one egg into each avocado half.
6. Sprinkle each egg with salt and black pepper and then, top evenly with the cheese.
7. Bake for about 12-15 minutes or until desired doneness of the egg whites.
8. Garnish with fresh chives and serve warm.

## Nutrition Values (Per Serving)

- Calories: 280
- Net Carbs: 2.4g
- Carbohydrate: 9.2g
- Fiber: 6.8g
- Protein: 8.5g
- Fat: 24.7g
- Sugar: 0.9g
- Sodium: 149mg

(**Tip:** To avoid the avocado halves from rolling and tipping over, make sure to position them against each other.)

# CHAPTER 2 | SOUPS & SALADS

## Chilled Cucumber Soup

**(Yields:** 2 servings / **Prep Time:** 15 minutes)

### Ingredients

- 1 cup English cucumber, peeled and chopped
- 1 scallion, chopped
- 2 tablespoons fresh parsley leaves
- 2 tablespoons fresh basil leaves
- ¼ teaspoon fresh lime zest, grated freshly
- 1 cup unsweetened coconut milk
- ¼ cup water
- ½ tablespoon fresh lime juice
- Salt and ground black pepper, as required

### Instructions

1. Add all the ingredients in a high-speed blender and pulse on high speed until smooth.
2. Transfer the soup into a large serving bowl.
3. Cover the bowl and refrigerate to chill for about 6 hours.
4. Serve chilled.

### Nutrition Values (Per Serving)

- Calories: 289
- Net Carbs: 5.6g
- Carbohydrate: 9g
- Fiber: 3.4g
- Protein: 3.4g
- Fat: 28.7g
- Sugar: 5.1g
- Sodium: 101mg

**(Tip:** You can replace the coconut milk with yogurt if you desired.)

## Chilled Avocado Soup

**(Yields:** 6 servings / **Prep Time:** 15 minutes)

### Ingredients

- 3 large avocados, peeled, pitted and roughly chopped
- 1/3 cup fresh cilantro leaves
- 3 cups homemade vegetable broth
- 2 tablespoons freshly squeezed lemon juice
- 1 teaspoon ground cumin
- ¼ teaspoon cayenne pepper
- Salt, to taste

## Instructions

1. Place all the ingredients in a high-speed blender and pulse on high speed until smooth.
2. Transfer the soup into a large serving bowl.
3. Cover the bowl and refrigerate to chill for at least 2-3 hours.
4. Serve chilled.

## Nutrition Values (Per Serving)

- Calories: 227
- Net Carbs: 2.6g
- Carbohydrate: 9.4g
- Fiber: 6.8g
- Protein: 4.5g
- Fat: 20.4g
- Sugar: 1g
- Sodium: 417mg

(**Tip:** Make sure to use ripe avocado for the best result.)

---

# Chilled Tomato Soup

(**Yields:** 5 servings / **Prep Time:** 15 minutes

## Ingredients

- 4-5 medium tomatoes, chopped
- 1½ cups cucumber, chopped
- ¾ cup onion, chopped
- ¼ cup fresh basil, chopped
- ¼ cup fresh parsley, chopped
- 2 tablespoons fresh lemon juice
- 1 tablespoon olive oil
- Salt and ground black pepper, as required

## Instructions

1. Place all the ingredients in a high-speed blender and pulse on high speed until smooth.
2. Transfer the soup into a large serving bowl.
3. Cover the bowl and refrigerate to chill for at least 1 hour.
4. Serve chilled.

## Nutrition Values (Per Serving)

- Calories: 56
- Net Carbs: 5g
- Carbohydrate: 6.9g
- Fiber: 1.9g
- Protein: 1.4g
- Fat: 3.1g
- Sugar: 4g
- Sodium: 40mg

# Chilled Strawberry Soup

**(Yields:** 6 servings / **Prep Time:** 20 minutes)

## Ingredients

- 1 pound fresh strawberries, hulled and sliced
- ½ of English cucumber, peeled, seeded and chopped
- ½ cup red bell pepper, seeded and chopped
- 1 tomato, roughly chopped
- ¼ of small jalapeño pepper, seeded and chopped
- 1 teaspoon fresh basil leaves
- 3 tablespoons olive oil
- 1 tablespoon balsamic vinegar
- Salt and ground black pepper, as required
- ½ cup homemade vegetable broth

## Instructions

1. In a high-speed blender, add all the ingredients except broth and pulse on high speed until smooth.
2. Transfer the soup into a large serving bowl.
3. Cover the bowl and refrigerate to chill for at least 6-8 hours.
4. Remove the bowl from refrigerator and stir in the broth until well combined.
5. Serve immediately.

## Nutrition Values (Per Serving)

- Calories: 97
- Net Carbs: 6g
- Carbohydrate: 8g
- Fiber: 2g
- Protein: 1.3g
- Fat: 7.4g
- Sugar: 5g
- Sodium: 93mg

# Green Veggies Soup

**(Yields:** 4 servings / **Prep Time:** 20 minutes / **Cooking Time:** 5 minutes)

## Ingredients

- ¼ cup almonds, soaked overnight and drained
- 1 large avocado, peeled, pitted and chopped
- 2 cups fresh spinach leaves
- 1 small zucchini, chopped
- 2 celery stalks, chopped
- ½ small green bell pepper, seeded and chopped
- 2 tablespoons onion, chopped
- 1 garlic clove, chopped
- ½ cup fresh cilantro leaves
- ¼ cup fresh parsley leaves
- 2 tablespoons fresh lemon juice
- Salt and ground black pepper, as required
- 1½ cups water

## Instructions

1. Add all the ingredients in a high-speed blender and pulse until smooth.
2. Transfer the soup into a pan and heat over medium-heat and cook for about 3-5 minutes or until heated through.
3. Serve immediately.

## Nutrition Values (Per Serving)

- Calories: 158
- Net Carbs: 4.3g
- Carbohydrate: 9.7g
- Fiber: 5.4g
- Protein: 3.5g
- Fat: 13g
- Sugar: 2.4g
- Sodium: 88mg

---

## Tomato & Basil Soup

**(Yields:** 8 servings / **Prep Time:** 15 minutes / **Cooking Time:** 28 minutes)

## Ingredients

- 3 tablespoons olive oil
- 2 small yellow onions, thinly sliced
- Salt, to taste
- 3 teaspoons curry powder
- 1 teaspoon ground cumin
- 1 teaspoon ground coriander
- ½ teaspoon red pepper flakes, crushed
- 1 (14-ounces) can sugar-free diced tomatoes with juice
- 1 (28-ounces) can sugar-free plum tomatoes with juices
- 5½ cups homemade vegetable broth
- ¼ cup fresh basil leaves, chopped

## Instructions

1. Heat the oil in a large Dutch oven over medium-low heat and cook the onion with one teaspoon of salt for about 10-12 minutes, stirring occasionally.
2. Stir in the spices and sauté for about 1 minute.
3. Add both cans of tomatoes alongside the juices, and broth and stir to combine.
4. Increase the heat to medium-high and cook until boiling.
5. Reduce the heat to medium-low and simmer for about 15 minutes.
6. Remove from the heat and with a hand blender, blend the soup until smooth.
7. Top with the fresh basil and serve.

### Nutrition Values (Per Serving)

- Calories: 113
- Net Carbs: 2.7g
- Carbohydrate: 9.4g
- Fiber: 6.7g
- Protein: 5.1g
- Fat: 6.7g
- Sugar: 5.5g
- Sodium: 553mg

---

## Yellow Squash Soup

**(Yields:** 6 servings / **Prep Time:** 20 minutes / **Cooking Time:** 35 minutes)

### Ingredients

- 2 tablespoons unsalted butter
- 2 yellow onions, chopped
- 6 garlic cloves, minced
- 6 cups yellow squash, seeded and cubed
- 4 thyme sprigs
- 4 cups homemade vegetable broth
- Salt and ground black pepper, as required
- 2 tablespoons fresh lemon juice
- 4 tablespoons Parmesan cheese, shredded
- 2 teaspoons fresh lemon peel, finely grated

### Instructions

1. Melt the butter in a large soup pan over medium heat and sauté the onions for about 5-6 minutes.
2. Stir in the garlic and sauté for about 1 minute.
3. Add the yellow squash cubes and cook for about 5 minutes.
4. Stir in the thyme, broth, salt, and black pepper and bring to a boil.
5. Reduce the heat to low and simmer, covered for about 15-20 minutes.
6. Remove the pan of soup from heat and discard the thyme sprigs.
7. Set the pan aside to cool slightly.
8. In a large blender, add the soup in batches and pulse until smooth.
9. Place soup into the same pan over medium heat.
10. Stir in the lemon juice and cook for about 2-3 minutes or until heated completely.
11. Garnish with Parmesan cheese and lemon peel.
12. Serve hot.

### Nutrition Values (Per Serving)

- Calories: 115
- Net Carbs: 7g
- Carbohydrate: 9.5g
- Fiber: 2.5g
- Protein: 6.6g
- Fat: 6g
- Sugar: 4.2g
- Sodium: 634mg

# Cauliflower Soup

**(Yields:** 5 servings / **Prep Time:** 15 minutes / **Cooking Time:** 25 minutes)

## Ingredients

- 2 tablespoons olive oil
- 1 small yellow onion, chopped
- 2 small carrots, peeled and chopped
- 2 small celery stalks, chopped
- 2 garlic cloves, minced
- 1 Serrano pepper, finely chopped
- 1 teaspoon ground turmeric
- 1 teaspoon ground coriander
- 1 teaspoon ground cumin
- ¼ teaspoon red pepper flakes, crushed
- 1 head cauliflower, chopped
- 4 cups homemade vegetable broth
- 1 cup unsweetened coconut milk
- 2 tablespoons freshly squeezed lime juice
- Salt and ground black pepper, as required
- 2 tablespoons fresh cilantro, finely chopped
- 1 teaspoon fresh lime zest, grated finely

## Instructions

1. In a large soup pan, heat the oil over medium heat and sauté the onion, carrot and celery for about 4 minutes.
2. Add the garlic, Serrano pepper and spices and sauté for about 1 minute.
3. Add the cauliflower and cook for about 5 minutes, stirring occasionally.
4. Add the broth and coconut milk and stir to combine.
5. Increase the heat to medium-high and bring to a boil.
6. Reduce the heat to low and simmer, partially covered for about 15 minutes.
7. Stir in the lime juice, salt, and black pepper and remove from the heat.
8. Serve hot with the topping of cilantro and lime zest.

## Nutrition Values (Per Serving)

- Calories: 121
- Net Carbs: 5.6g
- Carbohydrate: 8.3g
- Fiber: 2.7g
- Protein: 5.5g
- Fat: 7.7g
- Sugar: 3.6g
- Sodium: 676mg

---

# Mushroom Soup

**(Yields:** 4 servings / **Prep Time:** 15 minutes / **Cooking Time:** 20 minutes)

## Ingredients

- 3 tablespoons unsalted butter
- 1 scallion, sliced
- 1 garlic clove, crushed
- 5 cups fresh mushrooms, sliced

- 2 cups homemade vegetable broth
- Salt and ground black pepper, as required
- 1 cup heavy cream

## Instructions

1. Melt the butter in a large pan over medium heat and sauté the scallion and garlic for about 2-3 minutes.
2. Add the mushrooms and stir fry for about 5 minutes.
3. Stir in the broth and bring to a boil.
4. Cook for about 5 minutes.
5. Remove from the heat and with a stick blender, blend the soup until smooth.
6. Return the pan over medium heat.
7. Stir in the cream, salt, and black pepper and cook for about 2-3 minutes, stirring continuously.
8. Serve hot.

## Nutrition Values (Per Serving)

- Calories: 220
- Net Carbs: 3.7g
- Carbohydrate: 4.7g
- Fiber: 1g
- Protein: 6g
- Fat: 20.7g
- Sugar: 2g
- Sodium: 499mg

---

# Broccoli Soup

**(Yields:** 5 servings / **Prep Time:** 10 minutes / **Cooking Time:** 15 minutes)

## Ingredients

- 4 cups homemade chicken broth
- 20 ounces small broccoli florets
- 12 ounces cheddar cheese, cubed
- Salt and ground black pepper, as required
- 1 cup heavy cream

## Instructions

1. In a large soup pan, add the broth and broccoli over medium-high heat and bring to a boil.
2. Reduce the heat to low and simmer, covered for about 5-7 minutes.
3. Stir in the cheese and cook for about 2-3 minutes, stirring continuously.
4. Stir in the salt, black pepper, and cream and cook for about 2 minutes.
5. Serve hot.

### Nutrition Values (Per Serving)

- Calories: 426
- Net Carbs: 6g
- Carbohydrate: 9g
- Fiber: 3g
- Protein: 24.5g
- Fat: 32.9g
- Sugar: 2.9g
- Sodium: 1000mg

═══════════════════════════════════════════

## Bacon & Jalapeño Soup

**(Yields:** 5 servings / **Prep Time:** 15 minutes / **Cooking Time:** 22 minutes)

### Ingredients

- ¼ cup unsalted butter
- 4 medium jalapeño peppers, seeded and chopped
- 1 small yellow onion, chopped
- 1 teaspoon dried thyme, crushed
- ½ teaspoon ground cumin
- 3 cups homemade chicken broth
- 8 ounces cheddar cheese, shredded
- ¾ cup heavy cream
- Salt and ground black pepper, as required
- 6 cooked bacon slices, chopped

### Instructions

1. Melt 1 tablespoon of butter in a large pan over medium heat and sauté the jalapeño peppers for about 1-2 minutes.
2. With a slotted spoon, transfer the jalapeño peppers onto a plate.
3. In the same pan, melt the remaining butter over medium heat and sauté the onion for about 3-4 minutes.
4. Add the spices and sauté for about 1 minute.
5. Stir in the broth and bring to a boil.
6. Now, reduce the heat to low and cook for about 10 minutes.
7. Remove from the heat and with an immersion blender, blend until smooth.
8. Return the pan over medium-low heat.
9. Stir in ¾ of cooked bacon, cooked jalapeño, cheese, cream, salt, and black pepper and cook for about 5 minutes.
10. Top with the remaining bacon and serve hot.

### Nutrition Values (Per Serving)

- Calories: 549
- Net Carbs: 3.6g
- Carbohydrate: 4.5g
- Fiber: 0.9g
- Protein: 27.9g
- Fat: 46.5g
- Sugar: 1.7g
- Sodium: 1900mg

# Cheesy Chicken Soup

**(Yields:** 4 servings / **Prep Time:** 15 minutes / **Cooking Time:** 35 minutes)

## Ingredients

- 1 tablespoon butter
- 1¼ cups tomatoes, finely chopped
- 3 Serrano peppers, chopped
- 1 tablespoon taco seasoning
- 1 pound grass-fed skinless, boneless chicken breasts
- 3¼ cups homemade chicken broth
- 8 ounces, cream cheese, softened
- ½ cup heavy cream
- Salt, as required
- ¼ cup Monterrey Jack cheese, shredded

## Instructions

1. Melt the butter in a Dutch oven over medium heat and cook the tomatoes, Serrano and taco seasoning for about 1-2 minutes.
2. Add the chicken, and broth and bring to a boil.
3. Reduce the heat to medium-low and simmer, covered for about 25 minutes.
4. With a slotted spoon, transfer the chicken breasts onto a plate.
5. With 2 forks, shred the meat.
6. In the pan of soup, add the cream cheese, and cream and cook for about 2-3 minutes, stirring continuously.
7. Remove from the heat and with an immersion blender, blend the soup until smooth.
8. Return the pan over medium heat and stir in the shredded chicken and salt.
9. Cook for about 1-2 minutes.
10. Serve hot with the topping of cheese.

## Nutrition Values (Per Serving)

- Calories: 351
- Net Carbs: 4.3g
- Carbohydrate: 5.2g
- Fiber: 0.9g
- Protein: 47.5g
- Fat: 14.5g
- Sugar: 2.6g
- Sodium: 924mg

---

# Chicken & Salsa Soup

**(Yields:** 4 servings / **Prep Time:** 16 minutes / **Cooking Time:** 10 minutes)

## Ingredients

- ½ cup salsa verde
- 1 cup sharp cheddar cheese

- 4 ounces cream cheese, softened
- 2 cups homemade chicken broth
- 2 cups cooked grass-fed chicken, chopped

## Instructions

1. In a blender, add the salsa, cheddar cheese, cream cheese, and broth and pulse until smooth.
2. Transfer the mixture into a medium-sized pan over medium heat and cook for about 3-5 minutes or until heated through, stirring continuously.
3. Add the chicken and cook for about 3-5 minutes or until heated through, stirring frequently.
4. Serve warm.

## Nutrition Values (Per Serving)

- Calories: 345
- Net Carbs: 2.8g
- Carbohydrate: 2.9g
- Fiber: 0.1g
- Protein: 32.3g
- Fat: 22.1g
- Sugar: 1g
- Sodium: 857mg

# Chicken & Cauliflower Soup

**(Yields:** 4 servings / **Prep Time:** 20 minutes / **Cooking Time:** 25 minutes)

## Ingredients

- 2 tablespoons butter
- 1 medium carrot, peeled and chopped
- ½ cup yellow onion, chopped
- 2 celery stalks, chopped
- 1 garlic clove, minced
- 2 teaspoons xanthan gum
- 1 teaspoon dried parsley, crushed
- Salt and ground black pepper, as required
- 4 cups homemade chicken broth
- 10 ounces cauliflower, chopped
- 2 cups cooked grass-fed chicken, chopped
- 2 cups heavy cream
- ¼ cup fresh parsley, chopped

## Instructions

1. In a large soup pan, melt the butter over medium heat and sauté the carrot, onion and celery for about 3-4 minutes.
2. Add the garlic and sauté for about 1 minute.
3. Meanwhile, in a bowl, mix together the xanthan gum, parsley, salt and black pepper.

4. Stir in parsley mixture, broth and cauliflower in the pan and bring to a boil.
5. Reduce the heat to low and simmer, covered for about 15 minutes, stirring occasionally.
6. Stir in cooked chicken, cream, parsley, and salt and cook for about 4-5 minutes.
7. Serve hot.

## **Nutrition Values (Per Serving)**

- Calories: 442
- Net Carbs: 6.6g
- Carbohydrate: 11g
- Fiber: 4.4g
- Protein: 28.4g
- Fat: 31.6g
- Sugar: 4g
- Sodium: 986mg

---

## **Chicken & Mushroom Soup**

**(Yields:** 8 servings / **Prep Time:** 15 minutes / **Cooking Time:** 30 minutes)

## **Ingredients**

- 2 tablespoons unsalted butter
- 1 cup celery, chopped
- 1 large yellow onion, chopped
- 5-6 garlic cloves, minced
- 18 ounces mixed fresh mushrooms, sliced
- 1 teaspoon dried thyme, crushed
- 1 teaspoon fresh rosemary, chopped
- 1 pound grass-fed boneless, skinless chicken breasts
- 8 cups homemade chicken broth
- Salt and ground black pepper, as required
- 2/3 cup heavy cream
- 1 tablespoon arrowroot starch
- ¼ cup fresh parsley, chopped

## **Instructions**

1. In a large pan, melt the butter over medium heat and sauté the celery, onion and garlic for about 2-3 minutes.
2. Stir in the mushrooms, thyme, and rosemary and sauté for about 6-7 minutes.
3. Add the chicken breasts, broth, salt, and black pepper and bring to a boil.
4. Reduce the heat to low and simmer for about 15 minutes or until desired doneness of the chicken.
5. With a slotted spoon, transfer the chicken breasts onto a plate and cut into bite-sized pieces.
6. In a bowl, add the heavy cream and arrowroot starch and beat until smooth.
7. Add heavy cream mixture into the soup and stir to combine well.
8. Simmer for about 2-3 minutes or until desired thickness, stirring frequently.
9. Stir in the chopped chicken, parsley, salt, and pepper and remove from the heat.
10. Serve hot.

## Nutrition Values (Per Serving)

- Calories: 247
- Net Carbs: 5.5g
- Carbohydrate: 7.1g
- Fiber: 1.6g
- Protein: 24g
- Fat: 12.4g
- Sugar: 2.4g
- Sodium: 872mg

---

# Beef & Mushroom Soup

**(Yields:** 6 servings / **Prep Time:** 15 minutes / **Cooking Time:** 30 minutes)

## Ingredients

- 1¾ pounds grass-fed beef sirloin steaks, cut into thin strips
- ¼ cup butter
- 1 medium yellow onion, chopped
- 2 garlic cloves, minced
- 1 tablespoon Dijon mustard
- 2 teaspoons paprika
- 1¼ pounds white mushrooms, sliced
- 6 cups homemade chicken broth
- 1½ cups heavy whipping cream
- 3 tablespoons fresh lemon juice
- ¼ cup fresh parsley, chopped
- Salt and ground black pepper, as required

## Instructions

1. In a large pan, melt 2 tablespoons of butter over medium-high heat and sear the beef in 2 batches for about 3-4 minutes or until browned completely.
2. With a slotted spoon, transfer the beef slices into a bowl
3. In the same pan, melt the remaining butter over medium heat and sauté the onion and garlic for about 2-3 minutes.
4. Add the mushrooms and cook for about 3-4 minutes, stirring occasionally.
5. Stir in the cooked beef slices, Dijon mustard, paprika, and broth and bring to a boil.
6. Reduce the heat to low and cook for about 8-10 minutes.
7. Stir in the cream, salt and black pepper, and lemon juice and cook for about 1-2 minutes.
8. Garnish with parsley and serve hot.

## Nutrition Values (Per Serving)

- Calories: 491
- Net Carbs: 5.8g
- Carbohydrate: 7.6g
- Fiber: 1.8g
- Protein: 49.3g
- Fat: 29g
- Sugar: 1.6g
- Sodium: 160mg

# Beef Taco Soup

**(Yields:** 8 servings / **Prep Time:** 15 minutes / **Cooking Time:** 25 minutes)

## Ingredients

- 1 pound grass-fed ground beef
- ½ cup yellow onion, chopped
- 2 garlic cloves, minced
- 1 tablespoon ground cumin
- 1 teaspoon red chili powder
- 8 ounces cream cheese, softened
- 2 (10-ounces) cans sugar-free diced tomatoes and green chilies
- 7¼ cups homemade beef broth
- ½ cup heavy cream
- Salt, as required
- ½ cup fresh cilantro, chopped

## Instructions

1. Place a large pan over medium-high heat until heated.
2. Add the ground beef, onion, and garlic and cook for about 6-8 minutes, stirring frequently.
3. Drain the grease from pan.
4. In the pan, add the cumin, and chili powder and cook for about 2 minutes.
5. Stir in the cream cheese and cook for about 3-5 minutes, stirring continuously.
6. Stir in the tomatoes, broth, heavy cream, and salt and cook for about 10 minutes.
7. Garnish with cilantro and serve hot.

## Nutrition Values (Per Serving)

- Calories: 281
- Net Carbs: 4.7g
- Carbohydrate: 6g
- Fiber: 1.3g
- Protein: 19.2g
- Fat: 19.8g
- Sugar: 2.9g
- Sodium: 844mg

---

# Salmon Soup

**(Yields:** 4 servings / **Prep Time:** 20 minutes / **Cooking Time:** 20 minutes)

## Ingredients

- 1 tablespoon olive oil
- 1 yellow onion, chopped
- 1 garlic clove, minced
- 4 cups homemade chicken broth
- 1-pound boneless salmon, cubed
- 1 tablespoon low-sodium soy sauce
- 2 tablespoons fresh cilantro, chopped
- Ground black pepper, to taste
- 1 tablespoon fresh lime juice

## Instructions

1. Heat the oil in a large pan over medium heat and sauté the onion for about 5 minutes.
2. Add the garlic and sauté for about 1 minute.
3. Stir in the broth and bring to a boil over high heat.
4. Reduce the heat to low and simmer for about 10 minutes.
5. Add the salmon, and soy sauce and cook for about 3-4 minutes.
6. Stir in black pepper, lime juice, and cilantro and serve hot.

## Nutrition Values (Per Serving)

- Calories: 232
- Net Carbs: 3.5g
- Carbohydrate: 4.1g
- Fiber: 0.6g
- Protein: 27.5g
- Fat: 11.9g
- Sugar: 2.1g
- Sodium: 1000mg

(**Tip:** Make sure to use the low-sodium soy sauce.)

---

# Tilapia Soup

(**Yields:** 4 servings / **Prep Time:** 15 minutes / **Total Cooking Time:** 15 minutes)

## Ingredients

- 4 cups homemade chicken broth
- 1½ cups fresh spinach, chopped
- 10 fresh button mushrooms, sliced
- 4 (6-ounces) tilapia fillets, cut into bite-sized pieces
- 1 teaspoon red boat fish sauce
- 1 cup coconut cream
- Salt and ground black pepper, as required

## Instructions

1. In a large soup pan, add the broth over medium heat and bring to a boil.
2. Add vegetables and again bring to a boil.
3. Cook for about 3-4 minutes.
4. Stir in the tilapia and once again bring to a boil.
5. Cook for about 4 minutes.
6. Stir in the fish sauce, coconut cream, salt, and black pepper and cook for about 2-3 more minutes.
7. Remove from heat and serve hot.

### Nutrition Values (Per Serving)

- Calories: 330
- Net Carbs: 4.1g
- Carbohydrate: 6.1g
- Fiber: 2g
- Protein: 39.9g
- Fat: 17.4g
- Sugar: 3.5g
- Sodium: 1001mg

===

## Meatballs Soup

**(Yields:** 6 servings / **Prep Time:** 20 minutes / **Cooking Time:** 25 minutes)

### Ingredients

**For Turkey Meatballs:**

- 1 pound lean ground turkey
- 1 garlic clove, minced
- 1 organic egg, beaten
- ¼ cup Parmesan cheese, grated
- Salt and ground black pepper, as required

**For Soup:**

- 1 tablespoon olive oil
- 1 small yellow onion, finely chopped
- 1 garlic clove, minced
- 6 cups homemade chicken broth
- 7 cups fresh spinach, chopped
- Salt and ground black pepper, as required

### Instructions

1. For meatballs: in a bowl, add all the ingredients and mix until well combined.
2. Make 12 equal-sized small balls from the mixture.
3. In a large soup pan, heat oil over medium heat and sauté the onion for about 5-6 minutes.
4. Add the garlic and sauté for about 1 minute.
5. Stir in the broth and bring to a boil.
6. Carefully, place the balls in pan and bring to a boil.
7. Reduce the heat to low and simmer for about 10 minutes.
8. Stir in the spinach and bring soup to a gentle simmer.
9. Simmer for about 2-3 minutes.
10. Season with the salt and black pepper and serve hot.

### Nutrition Values (Per Serving)

- Calories: 203
- Net Carbs: 2.7g
- Carbohydrate: 3.7g
- Fiber: 1g
- Protein: 23.1g
- Fat: 10.8g
- Sugar: 1.4g
- Sodium: 915mg

# Berries & Spinach Salad

**(Yields:** 4 servings / **Prep Time:** 15 minutes)

## Ingredients

**For Salad:**

- 8 ounces fresh baby spinach
- ¾ cup fresh strawberries, hulled and sliced
- ¾ cup fresh blueberries
- ¼ cup feta cheese, crumbled

**For Dressing:**

- 1/3 cup olive oil
- 2 tablespoons fresh lemon juice
- ¼ teaspoon liquid stevia
- 1/8 teaspoon paprika
- 1/8 teaspoon garlic powder
- Salt, as required

## Instructions

1. For salad: in a bowl, mix together the spinach, berries and almonds.
2. For dressing: in another small bowl, add all the ingredients and beat until well combined.
3. Place the dressing over salad and gently, toss to coat well.
4. Serve immediately.

## Nutrition Values (Per Serving)

- Calories: 208
- Net Carbs: 8.6g
- Carbohydrate: 11.1g
- Fiber: 2.5g
- Protein: 3.4g
- Fat: 19.3g
- Sugar: 4.8g
- Sodium: 190mg

**(Tip:** You can use berries of your choice)

---

# Cabbage Salad

**(Yields:** 6 servings / **Prep Time:** 15 minutes)

## Ingredients

**For Salad:**

- 4 cups green cabbage, shredded
- ¼ onion, thinly sliced
- 1 teaspoon lime zest, grated freshly
- 3 tablespoons fresh cilantro, chopped

**For Dressing:**

- ¾ cup mayonnaise
- 2 teaspoons fresh lime juice
- 2 teaspoons chili sauce
- ½ teaspoon Erythritol
- 2 garlic cloves, minced

## Instructions

1. For salad: in a bowl, mix together the cabbage, onion, lime zest and cilantro.
2. For dressing: in another small bowl, add all the ingredients and beat until well combined.
3. Place the dressing over salad and gently, toss to coat well.
4. Cover and refrigerate to chill before serving.

## Nutrition Values (Per Serving)

- Calories: 196
- Net Carbs: 2.3g
- Carbohydrate: 3.6g
- Fiber: 1.3g
- Protein: 0.7g
- Fat: 20.1g
- Sugar: 1.7g
- Sodium: 231mg

**(Tip:** You can preserve this salad into mason jars in your refrigerator for about 1 day.)

---

# Cucumber & Spinach Salad

**(Yields:** 6 servings / **Prep Time:** 15 minutes)

## Ingredients

**For Dressing:**

- 5 tablespoons olive oil
- 4 tablespoons plain Greek yogurt
- 2 tablespoons fresh lemon juice
- 2 tablespoons fresh mint leaves, finely chopped
- 1 teaspoon Erythritol
- Salt and ground black pepper, as required

**For Salad:**

- 3 cups cucumbers, peeled, seeded and sliced
- 10 cups fresh baby spinach
- ¼ of medium yellow onion, sliced

## Instructions

1. For dressing: add all the ingredients in a bowl and beat until well combined.
2. Cover and refrigerate to chill for about 1 hour.
3. In a large serving bowl, mix together all the salad ingredients.
4. Place dressing over salad and toss to coat well.
5. Serve immediately.

## Nutrition Values (Per Serving)

- Calories: 130
- Net Carbs: 3.5g
- Carbohydrate: 5.1g
- Fiber: 1.6g
- Protein: 2.5g
- Fat: 12.1g
- Sugar: 2.1g
- Sodium: 77mg

# Broccoli Salad

**(Yields:** 4 servings / **Prep Time:** 15 minutes)

## Ingredients

**For Salad:**

- 8 cups small fresh broccoli florets
- 1 (8-ounces) package Colby-Monterey Jack cheese, cubed
- 2 cups fresh strawberries, hulled and sliced
- ¼ cup fresh mint leaves, chopped

**For Dressing:**

- 1 cup mayonnaise
- 1 teaspoon balsamic vinegar
- 2 teaspoons Erythritol
- Salt and ground black pepper, as required

## Instructions

1. For salad: in a large serving bowl, add all the ingredients and mix well.
2. For the dressing: in another bowl, add all the ingredients and beat until well combined.
3. Place the dressing over salad and gently, stir to combine.
4. Serve immediately.

## Nutrition Values (Per Serving)

- Calories: 374
- Net Carbs: 6.2g
- Carbohydrate: 11g
- Fiber: 4.8g
- Protein: 6.3g
- Fat: 35.2g
- Sugar: 4.1g
- Sodium: 184mg

**(Tip:** You can use cheddar or Gouda cheese instead of Colby-Monterey Jack cheese.)

---

# Tomato & Mozzarella Salad

**(Yields:** 6 servings / **Prep Time:** 15 minutes)

## Ingredients

- 4 cups cherry tomatoes, halved
- 1½ pounds mozzarella cheese, cubed
- ¼ cup fresh basil leaves, chopped
- ¼ cup olive oil
- 2 tablespoons fresh lemon juice
- 1 teaspoon fresh oregano, minced
- 1 teaspoon fresh parsley, minced
- 2-4 drops liquid stevia
- Salt and ground black pepper, as required

## Instructions

1. In a salad bowl, mix together the tomatoes, mozzarella and basil.
2. In another small bowl, place the remaining ingredients and beat until well combined.
3. Place dressing over salad and toss to coat well.
4. Serve immediately.

## Nutrition Values (Per Serving)

- Calories: 116
- Net Carbs: 3.6g
- Carbohydrate: 5.2g
- Fiber: 1.6g
- Protein: 3.2g
- Fat: 10g
- Sugar: 3.3g
- Sodium: 77mg

---

# Mixed Veggie Salad

**(Yields:** 4 servings / **Prep Time:** 20 minutes)

## Ingredients

**For Dressing:**

- 1 small avocado, peeled, pitted and chopped
- ¼ cup plain Greek yogurt
- 1 small yellow onion, chopped
- 1 garlic clove, chopped
- 2 tablespoons fresh parsley
- 2 tablespoons fresh lemon juice

**For Salad:**

- 6 cups fresh spinach, shredded
- 2 medium zucchinis, cut into thin slices
- ½ cup celery, sliced
- ½ cup red bell pepper, seeded and thinly sliced
- ½ cup yellow onion, thinly sliced
- ½ cup cucumber, thinly sliced
- ½ cup cherry tomatoes, halved
- ¼ cup Kalamata olives, pitted
- ½ cup feta cheese, crumbled

## Instructions

1. For dressing: in a food processor, add all the ingredients and pulse until smooth.
2. For the salad: in a salad bowl, add all the ingredients and mix well.
3. Place the dressing over salad and gently, toss to coat well.
4. Serve immediately.

### Nutrition Values (Per Serving)

- Calories: 148
- Net Carbs: 6.3g
- Carbohydrate: 10.9g
- Fiber: 4.6g
- Protein: 5.3g
- Fat: 10.3g
- Sugar: 4.4g
- Sodium: 238mg

---

## Creamy Shrimp Salad

**(Yields:** 12 servings / **Prep Time:** 20 minutes / **Cooking Time:** 3 minutes)

### Ingredients

- 4 pounds large shrimp
- 1 lemon, quartered
- 3 cups celery stalks, chopped
- 1 yellow onion, chopped
- 2 cups mayonnaise
- 2 tablespoons fresh lemon juice
- 1 teaspoon Dijon mustard
- Salt and ground black pepper, as required

### Instructions

1. In a pan of lightly salted boiling water, add the shrimp, and lemon and cook for about 3 minutes.
2. Drain the shrimps well and let them cool.
3. Then, peel and devein the shrimps.
4. In a large bowl, add the cooked shrimp and remaining ingredients and gently, stir to combine.
5. Serve immediately.

### Nutrition Values (Per Serving)

- Calories: 429
- Net Carbs: 3.4g
- Carbohydrate: 4.1g
- Fiber: 0.7g
- Protein: 34.8g
- Fat: 29.3g
- Sugar: 0.8g
- Sodium: 648mg

---

## Shrimp & Green Beans Salad

**(Yields:** 4 servings / **Prep Time:** 20 minutes / **Cooking Time:** 8 minutes)

### Ingredients

**For Shrimp:**

- 2 tablespoons olive oil
- 2 tablespoons fresh key lime juice
- 4 large garlic cloves, peeled
- 2 sprigs fresh rosemary leaves
- ½ teaspoon garlic salt
- 20 large shrimp, peeled and deveined

**For Salad:**

- 1 pound fresh green beans, trimmed
- ¼ cup olive oil
- 1 onion, sliced
- Salt and ground black pepper, as required
- ½ cup garlic and herb feta cheese, crumbled

## Instructions

1. For shrimp marinade: in a blender, add all the ingredients except shrimp and pulse until smooth.
2. Transfer the marinade in a large bowl.
3. Place the shrimp and generously mix with marinade.
4. Cover the bowl and refrigerate to marinate for at least 30 minutes.
5. Preheat the broiler of oven. Arrange the rack in top position of oven. Line a large baking sheet with a piece of foil.
6. Place shrimp with marinade onto the prepared baking sheet.
7. Broil for about 3-4 minutes per side.
8. Transfer the shrimp mixture into a bowl and refrigerate until using.
9. Meanwhile, for the salad: in a pan of salted boiling water, add the green beans and cook for about 3-4 minutes.
10. Drain the green beans well and rinse under cold running water.
11. Transfer the green beans into a large bowl.
12. Add the oil, onion, shrimp, salt and black pepper and stir to combine.
13. Cover and refrigerate to chill for about 1 hour.
14. Stir in the cheese just before serving.

## Nutrition Values (Per Serving)

- Calories: 303
- Net Carbs: 6.5g
- Carbohydrate: 10.5g
- Fiber: 4g
- Protein: 24.3g
- Fat: 18.5g
- Sugar: 2.5g
- Sodium: 100mg

---

# Salmon Salad

**(Yields:** 8 servings / **Prep Time:** 15 minutes)

## Ingredients

- 12 hard-boiled organic eggs, peeled and cubed
- 1 pound smoked salmon, chopped
- 3 celery stalks, chopped
- 1 yellow onion, chopped
- 4 tablespoons fresh dill, chopped
- 2 cups mayonnaise
- Salt and ground black pepper, as required
- 8 cups fresh lettuce leaves

## Instructions

1. In a large serving bowl, add all the ingredients except lettuce leaves and gently stir to combine.
2. Cover and refrigerate to chill before serving.
3. Divide the lettuce onto serving plates and top with salmon salad.
4. Serve immediately.

## Nutrition Values (Per Serving)

- Calories: 547
- Net Carbs: 2.5g
- Carbohydrate: 3.5g
- Fiber: 1g
- Protein: 20.1g
- Fat: 50.3g
- Sugar: 1.7g
- Sodium: 509mg

# Lobster Salad

**(Yields:** 14 servings / **Prep Time:** 15 minutes)

## Ingredients

- 5 pounds cooked lobster meat, shredded
- 3 yellow bell peppers, seeded and chopped
- 6 celery stalks, chopped
- 1 large yellow onion, chopped
- 2 cups mayonnaise
- Freshly ground black pepper, as required

## Instructions

1. In a salad bowl, add all the ingredients and mix until well combined.
2. Refrigerate to chill before serving.

## Nutrition Values (Per Serving)

- Calories: 364
- Net Carbs: 2.5g
- Carbohydrate: 3.2g
- Fiber: 0.7g
- Protein: 31.2g
- Fat: 24.3g
- Sugar: 1.8g
- Sodium: 1000mg

# Tuna Salad

**(Yields:** 3 servings / **Prep Time:** 20 minutes)

## Ingredients

- 2 (6-ounces) cans water packed solid white tuna, drained
- ¼ cup fresh cranberries
- 3 tablespoons mayonnaise
- 1/3 teaspoon dried dill weed

## Instructions

1. In a large salad bowl, place the tuna and with a fork, mash it completely.
2. Add the remaining ingredients and stir to mix well.
3. Serve immediately.

## Nutrition Values (Per Serving)

- Calories: 1274
- Net Carbs: 4.1g
- Carbohydrate: 4.4g
- Fiber: 0.3g
- Protein: 30.2g
- Fat: 14.1g
- Sugar: 1.3g
- Sodium: 161mg

---

# Crab Salad

**(Yields:** 4 servings / **Prep Time:** 15 minutes)

## Ingredients

- 1 pound jumbo lump crabmeat, picked over
- 1 celery stalk, peeled, and cut into 1/8-inch pieces
- 4 teaspoons fresh chives, minced
- 1 teaspoon fresh tarragon leaves, minced
- 1/3 cup mayonnaise
- 2 tablespoons sour cream
- 1 teaspoon fresh lemon juice
- ½ teaspoon Dijon mustard
- Salt and ground black pepper, as required

## Instructions

1. In a bowl, add the crabmeat, celery, chives, and tarragon and toss to coat well.
2. In another bowl, mix well mayonnaise, sour cream, lemon juice, mustard, salt and black pepper.
3. Place the dressing into bowl of crabmeat mixture and gently, stir to combine.
4. Serve immediately.

## Nutrition Values (Per Serving)

- Calories: 236
- Net Carbs: 2.5g
- Carbohydrate: 2.6g
- Fiber: 0.1g
- Protein: 14.5g
- Fat: 16.7g
- Sugar: 0.1g
- Sodium: 882mg

---

# Beef Salad

**(Yields:** 6 servings / **Prep Time:** 215 minutes / **Cooking Time:** 10 minutes)

## Ingredients

- 1 pound grass-fed ground beef
- 1 teaspoon olive oil
- 1 tablespoon taco seasoning
- 8 ounces Romaine lettuce, chopped
- 1 1/3 cups grape tomatoes, halved
- 1 large cucumber, chopped
- ½ cup scallions, chopped
- ¾ cup Cheddar cheese, shredded
- 1/3 cup salsa
- 1/3 cup sour cream

## Instructions

1. In a skillet, heat the oil over high heat and stir fry beef for about 8-10 minutes, breaking up the beef with a spatula.
2. Stir in the taco seasoning and remove from heat.
3. Set aside to cool slightly.
4. Meanwhile, in a large bowl, add the remaining ingredients and mix until well combined.
5. Add the ground beef and toss to coat well.
6. Serve immediately.

## Nutrition Values (Per Serving)

- Calories: 256
- Net Carbs: 6.1g
- Carbohydrate: 7.5g
- Fiber: 1.4g
- Protein: 20.5g
- Fat: 15.7g
- Sugar: 3.2g
- Sodium: 343mg

# Turkey Salad

**(Yields:** 6 servings / **Prep Time:** 20 minutes / **Cooking Time:** 13 minutes)

## Ingredients

- 1 pound ground turkey
- 1 tablespoon olive oil
- Salt and ground black pepper, as required
- ¼ cup water
- ½ of English cucumber, chopped
- 4 cups green cabbage, shredded
- ½ cup fresh mint leaves, chopped
- 2 tablespoons fresh lime juice
- ¼ cup walnuts, chopped

## Instructions

1. Heat the oil in a skillet over medium-high heat and cook the turkey for about 6-8 minutes, breaking up the meat with a spatula.
2. Stir in the salt, black pepper, and water and cook for about 4-5 minutes or until almost all the liquid is evaporated.
3. Remove from heat and transfer the turkey into a bowl.
4. Set the bowl aside to cool completely.
5. In a large serving bowl, mix well vegetables, mint and lime juice.
6. Add the cooked turkey and stir to combine.
7. Top with the chopped walnuts and serve.

## Nutrition Values (Per Serving)

- Calories: 219
- Net Carbs: 2.6g
- Carbohydrate: 4.8g
- Fiber: 2.2g
- Protein: 22.9g
- Fat: 13.8g
- Sugar: 2g
- Sodium: 120mg

# Chicken Salad

(**Yields:** 8 servings / **Prep Time:** 20 minutes / **Cooking Time:** 16 minutes)

## Ingredients

- 2 pounds grass-fed boneless, skinless chicken breasts
- ½ cup olive oil
- ¼ cup fresh lemon juice
- 2 tablespoons Erythritol
- 1 garlic clove, minced
- Salt and ground black pepper, as required
- 4 cups fresh strawberries, hulled and sliced
- 8 cups fresh spinach, torn

## Instructions

1. For marinade: in a large bowl, add the oil, lemon juice, Erythritol, garlic, salt, and black pepper and beat until well combined.
2. Place chicken and ¾ cup marinade in a large resealable plastic bag.
3. Seal bag and shake to coat well.
4. Refrigerate overnight.
5. Cover the bowl of remaining marinade and refrigerate before serving.
6. Preheat the grill to medium heat. Grease the grill grate.
7. Remove the chicken from bag and discard the marinade.
8. Place the chicken onto grill grate and grill, covered for about 5-8 minutes per side.
9. Remove the chicken from grill and cut into bite sized pieces.
10. In a large bowl, mix together the chicken pieces, strawberries and spinach.
11. Add the reserved marinade and toss to coat.
12. Serve immediately.

## Nutrition Values (Per Serving)

- Calories: 356
- Net Carbs: 4g
- Carbohydrate: 6.1g
- Fiber: 2.1g
- Protein: 34.2g
- Fat: 21.4g
- Sugar: 3.8g
- Sodium: 143mg

# CHAPTER 3 | BEEF & LAMB

## Beef Curry

**(Yields:** 8 servings / **Prep Time:** 10 minutes / **Cooking Time:** 3 hours 10 minutes)

## Ingredients

- 2 tablespoons butter
- 3 tablespoons Thai red curry paste with no added sugar
- 2½ cups unsweetened coconut milk
- ½ cup homemade chicken broth
- 2½ pounds grass-fed beef chuck roast, cubed into 1-inch size
- Salt and ground black pepper, as required
- ¼ cup fresh cilantro, chopped

## Instructions

1. Melt the butter in a large pan over low heat and sauté the curry paste for about 4-5 minutes.
2. Stir in the coconut milk, and broth and bring to a gentle simmer, stirring occasionally.
3. Simmer for about 4-5 minutes.
4. Stir in beef and bring to a boil over medium heat.
5. Adjust the heat to low and cook, covered for about 2½ hours, stirring occasionally
6. Remove from heat and with a slotted spoon, transfer the beef into a bowl.
7. Set the pan of curry aside for about 10 minutes.
8. With a slotted spoon, remove the fats from top of curry.
9. Return the pan over medium heat.
10. Stir in the cooked beef and bring to a gentle simmer.
11. Adjust the heat to low and cook, uncovered for about 30 minutes or until desired thickness.
12. Stir in salt and black pepper and remove from the heat.
13. Garnish with fresh cilantro and serve hot.

## Nutrition Values (Per Serving)

- Calories: 753
- Net Carbs: 4.1g
- Carbohydrate: 5.8g
- Fiber: 1.7g
- Protein: 39.4g
- Fat: 63.6g
- Sugar: 2.6g
- Sodium: 190mg

**(Tip:** For the best result, cut the beef into equal-sized cubes.)

# Spicy Steak Curry

**(Yields:** 6 servings / **Prep Time:** 15 minutes / **Cooking Time:** 40 minutes)

## Ingredients

- 1 cup plain yogurt
- ½ teaspoon garlic paste
- ½ teaspoon ginger paste
- ½ teaspoon ground cloves
- ½ teaspoon ground cumin
- 2 teaspoons red pepper flakes, crushed
- ¼ teaspoon ground turmeric
- Salt, to taste
- 2 pounds grass-fed round steak, cut into pieces
- ¼ cup olive oil
- 1 medium yellow onion, thinly sliced
- 1½ tablespoons fresh lemon juice
- ¼ cup fresh cilantro, chopped

## Instructions

1. In a large bowl, mix well yogurt, garlic paste, ginger paste and spices.
2. Add the steak pieces and generously coat with the yogurt mixture.
3. Set aside for at least 15 minutes.
4. Heat the oil in a large skillet over medium-high heat and sauté the onion for about 4-5 minutes.
5. Add the steak pieces with marinade and stir to combine.
6. Immediately, adjust the heat to low and simmer, covered and cook for about 25 minutes, stirring occasionally.
7. Stir in the lemon juice and simmer for about 10 more minutes.
8. Garnish with fresh cilantro and serve hot.

## Nutrition Values (Per Serving)

- Calories: 440
- Net Carbs: 4.8g
- Carbohydrate: 5.5g
- Fiber: 0.7g
- Protein: 48.3g
- Fat: 23.7g
- Sugar: 3.8g
- Sodium: 149mg

---

# Beef Stew

**(Yields:** 4 servings / **Prep Time:** 15 minutes / **Cooking Time:** 1 hour 40 minutes)

## Ingredients

- 1 1/3 pounds grass-fed chuck roast, trimmed and cubed into 1-inch size
- Salt and ground black pepper, as required
- 2 tablespoons butter
- 1 yellow onion, finely chopped
- 2 garlic cloves, finely chopped
- 1 cup homemade beef broth

- 1 bay leaf
- ½ teaspoon dried thyme, crushed
- ½ teaspoon dried rosemary, crushed
- 1 carrot, peeled and thinly sliced
- 4 ounces celery stalks, thinly sliced
- 1 tablespoon fresh lemon juice

## Instructions

1. Sprinkle the beef cubes with salt and black pepper.
2. Melt the butter in a Dutch oven over medium-high heat and sear the beef cubes for about 4-5 minutes.
3. Add the onion and garlic and stir to combine.
4. Adjust the heat to medium and cook for about 4-5 minutes.
5. Add the broth, bay leaf and dried herbs and bring to a boil.
6. Lower the heat to medium-low and simmer for about 45 minutes.
7. Stir in the carrot and celery and simmer for about 30-45 minutes.
8. Stir in lemon juice, salt, and black pepper and remove from the heat.
9. Serve hot.

## Nutrition Values (Per Serving)

- Calories: 413
- Net Carbs: 4.3g
- Carbohydrate: 5.9g
- Fiber: 1.6g
- Protein: 52g
- Fat: 3.18.8g
- Sugar: 2.6g
- Sodium: 406mg

---

# Beef & Cabbage Stew

**(Yields:** 8 servings / **Prep Time:** 15 minutes / **Cooking Time:** 2 hours 10 minutes)

## Ingredients

- 2 pounds grass-fed beef stew meat, trimmed and cubed into 1-inch size
- 1 1/3 cups homemade hot chicken broth
- 2 yellow onions, chopped
- 2 bay leaves
- 1 teaspoon Greek seasoning
- Salt and ground black pepper, as required
- 3 celery stalks, chopped
- 1 (8-ounces) package shredded cabbage
- 1 (6-ounces) can sugar-free tomato sauce
- 1 (8-ounces) can sugar-free whole plum tomatoes, roughly chopped with liquid

## Instructions

1. Heat a large nonstick pan over medium-high heat and sear the beef for about 4-5 minutes or until browned.

2. Stir in the broth, onion, bay leaves, Greek seasoning, salt, and black pepper and bring to a boil.
3. Adjust the heat to low and cook, covered for about 1¼ hours.
4. Stir in the celery, and cabbage and cook, covered for about 30 minutes.
5. Stir in the tomato sauce and chopped plum tomatoes and cook, uncovered for about 15-20 minutes.
6. Stir in the salt and remove from heat.
7. Discard bay leaves and serve hot.

## Nutrition Values (Per Serving)

- Calories: 247
- Net Carbs: 4.9g
- Carbohydrate: 7g
- Fiber: 2.1g
- Protein: 36.5g
- Fat: 7.5g
- Sugar: 3.9g
- Sodium: 346mg

---

# Beef & Mushroom Chili

**(Yields:** 8 servings / **Prep Time:** 15 minutes / **Cooking Time:** 3 hours 10 minutes)

## Ingredients

- 2 pounds grass-fed ground beef
- 1 yellow onion, chopped
- ½ cup green bell pepper, seeded and chopped
- ½ cup carrot, peeled and chopped
- 4 ounces fresh mushrooms, sliced
- 2 garlic cloves, minced
- 1 (6-ounces) can sugar-free tomato paste
- 2 tablespoons red chili powder
- 1 tablespoon ground cumin
- 1 teaspoon ground cinnamon
- 1 teaspoon red pepper flakes, crushed
- ½ teaspoon ground allspice
- Salt and ground black pepper, as required
- 4 cups water
- ½ cup sour cream

## Instructions

1. Heat a large nonstick pan over medium-high heat and cook the beef for about 8-10 minutes.
2. Drain the excess grease from pan.
3. Stir in the remaining ingredients except sour cream and bring to a boil.
4. Adjust the heat to low and cook, covered for about 3 hours.
5. Top with sour cream and serve hot.

## Nutrition Values (Per Serving)

- Calories: 246
- Net Carbs: 5.9g
- Carbohydrate: 8.2g
- Fiber: 2.3g
- Protein: 25.1g
- Fat: 12.4g
- Sugar: 3.5g
- Sodium: 143mg

# Beef with Mushroom Gravy

**(Yields:** 4 servings / **Prep Time:** 15 minutes / **Cooking Time:** 28 minutes)

## Ingredients

**For Mushroom Gravy:**

- 4 bacon slices, chopped
- 3 tablespoons butter
- 3 garlic cloves, minced
- 1 teaspoon dried thyme
- 1½ cups fresh button mushrooms, sliced
- Salt and ground black pepper, as required
- 7 ounces cream cheese, softened
- ½ cup heavy cream

**For Steak:**

- 4 (6-ounces) grass-fed beef tenderloin filets
- Salt and ground black pepper, as required
- 3 tablespoons butter

## Instructions

1. For mushroom gravy: heat a large nonstick skillet over medium-high heat and cook the bacon for about 8-10 minutes.
2. With a slotted spoon, transfer the bacon onto a paper towel-lined plate to drain.
3. Discard the bacon grease from skillet.
4. In the same skillet, melt butter over medium heat and sauté the garlic and thyme for about 1 minute.
5. Stir in the mushrooms, salt, and black pepper and cook for about 5-7 minutes, stirring frequently.
6. Adjust the heat to low and stir in the cream cheese until smooth.
7. Stir in cream and cook for about 2-3 minutes or until heated completely.
8. Meanwhile, rub the beef filets evenly with salt and black pepper.
9. In a large cast iron skillet, melt the butter over medium heat and cook the filets for about 5-7 minutes per side.
10. Remove the skillet of mushroom gravy from heat and stir in the bacon.
11. Place the filets onto serving plates and serve with the topping of mushroom gravy.

## Nutrition Values (Per Serving)

- Calories: 895
- Net Carbs: 3.5g
- Carbohydrate: 3.9g
- Fiber: 0.4g
- Protein: 65.2g
- Fat: 67.9g
- Sugar: 0.6g
- Sodium: 1048mg

**(Tip:** You can use mushroom of your choice.)

# Steak with Cheese Sauce

**(Yields:** 4 servings / **Prep Time:** 15 minutes / **Cooking Time:** 17 minutes)

## Ingredients

- 18 ounces grass-fed filet mignon, cut into thin steaks
- Salt and ground black pepper, as required
- 2 tablespoons butter
- ½ cup yellow onion, shredded
- 5¼ ounces blue cheese, cubed
- 1 cup heavy cream
- 1 garlic clove, minced
- Pinch of ground nutmeg

## Instructions

1. Melt the butter in a pan over medium heat and cook onion for about 5-8 minutes, stirring frequently.
2. Add the blue cheese, heavy cream, garlic, nutmeg, salt, and black pepper and stir to combine.
3. Adjust the heat to medium-low and cook for about 3-5 minutes, stirring continuously.
4. Meanwhile, sprinkle the filet mignon steaks with salt and black pepper.
5. Heat a lightly greased grill pan over high heat and cook the steaks for about 4 minutes per side.
6. Transfer the steaks onto a plate and set aside.
7. Divide the steaks onto serving plates and top with cheese sauce.
8. Serve immediately.

## Nutrition Values (Per Serving)

- Calories: 521
- Net Carbs: 3g
- Carbohydrate: 3.3g
- Fiber: 0.3g
- Protein: 44.7g
- Fat: 36g
- Sugar: 0.9g
- Sodium: 686mg

---

# Steak with Blueberry Sauce

**(Yields:** 4 servings / **Prep Time:** 15 minutes / **Cooking Time:** 20 minutes)

## Ingredients

**For Sauce:**

- 2 tablespoons butter
- 2 tablespoons yellow onion, chopped
- 2 garlic cloves, minced
- 1 teaspoon fresh thyme, finely chopped
- 1 1/3 cups homemade beef broth
- 2 tablespoons fresh lemon juice
- ¾ cup fresh blueberries

**For Steak:**
- 2 tablespoons butter
- 4 (6-ounces) grass-fed flank steaks
- Salt and ground black pepper, as required

## Instructions

1. For sauce: in a pan, melt butter over medium heat and sauté the onion for about 2-3 minutes.
2. Add the garlic, and thyme and sauté for about 1 minute.
3. Stir in the broth and bring to a gentle simmer.
4. Adjust the heat to low and cook for about 10 minutes.
5. Meanwhile, for the steak: season it with salt and black pepper.
6. In a skillet, melt the butter over medium-high heat and cook steaks for about 3-4 minutes per side.
7. With a slotted spoon, transfer the steak onto serving plates.
8. Add sauce in the skillet and stir to scrape up brown bits from the bottom.
9. Stir in the lemon juice, blueberries, salt, and black pepper and cook for about 1-2 minutes.
10. Remove from heat and place blueberry sauce over the steaks.
11. Serve immediately.

## Nutrition Values (Per Serving)

- Calories: 467
- Net Carbs: 4.6g
- Carbohydrate: 5.5g
- Fiber: 0.9g
- Protein: 49.5g
- Fat: 3.3g
- Sugar: 1.6g
- Sodium: 473mg

---

# Grilled Steak

**(Yields:** 6 servings / **Prep Time:** 15 minutes / **Cooking Time:** 12 minutes)

## Ingredients

- 1 teaspoon fresh lemon zest, finely grated
- 1 garlic clove, minced
- 1 tablespoon red chili powder
- 1 tablespoon paprika
- 1 tablespoon ground coffee
- Salt and ground black pepper, as required
- 2 (1½-pounds) grass-fed skirt steaks

### Instructions

1. In a bowl, add all the ingredients except steaks and mix until well combined.
2. Generously rub the steaks with spice mixture and keep aside for about 30-40 minutes.
3. Preheat the grill to high heat. Grease the grill grate.
4. Grill the steaks for about 5-6 minutes per side or until desired doneness.
5. Remove from the grill and place onto a cutting board for about 5-10 minutes before slicing.
6. With a sharp knife, cut the steaks into desired size slices and serve.

### Nutrition Values (Per Serving)

- Calories: 473
- Net Carbs: 0.7g
- Carbohydrate: 1.6g
- Fiber: 0.9g
- Protein: 60.8g
- Fat: 32.2g
- Sugar: 0.2g
- Sodium: 213mg

(**Tip:** Don't forget to properly clean the grill and grease before cooking.)

---

## Roasted Tenderloin

(**Yields:** 10 servings / **Prep Time:** 10 minutes / **Cooking Time:** 50 minutes)

### Ingredients

- 1 (3-pounds) grass-fed center-cut beef tenderloin roast
- 4 garlic cloves, minced
- 1 tablespoon fresh rosemary, minced and divided
- Salt and ground black pepper, as required
- 1 tablespoon olive oil

### Instructions

1. Preheat the oven to 425 degrees F. Grease a large shallow roasting pan.
2. Place beef into the prepared roasting pan.
3. Rub the beef with garlic, rosemary, salt, and black pepper and drizzle with oil.
4. Roast the beef for about 45-50 minutes.
5. Remove from oven and place the roast onto a cutting board for about 10 minutes.
6. With a sharp knife, cut the beef tenderloin into desired size slices and serve.

### Nutrition Values (Per Serving)

- Calories: 295
- Net Carbs: 0.4g
- Carbohydrate: 0.6g
- Fiber: 0.2g
- Protein: 39.5g
- Fat: 13.9g
- Sugar: 0g
- Sodium: 96mg

# Garlicky Prime Rib Roast

**(Yields:** 15 servings / **Prep Time:** 15 minutes / **Cooking Time:** 1 hour 35 minutes**)**

## Ingredients

- 10 garlic cloves, minced
- 2 teaspoons dried thyme, crushed
- 2 tablespoons olive oil
- Salt and ground black pepper, as required
- 1 (10-pounds) grass-fed prime rib roast

## Instructions

1. In a bowl, add the garlic, thyme, oil, salt, and black pepper and mix until well combined.
2. Coat the rib roast evenly with garlic mixture and arrange in a large roasting pan, fatty side up.
3. Set aside to marinate at the room temperature for at least 1 hour.
4. Preheat the oven to 500 degrees F.
5. Place the roasting pan into oven and roast for about 20 minutes.
6. Now, reduce the temperature to 325 degrees F and roast for about 65-75 minutes.
7. Remove from oven and place the rib roast onto a cutting board for about 10-15 minutes before slicing.
8. With a sharp knife, cut the rib roast into desired size slices and serve.

## Nutrition Values (Per Serving)

- Calories: 499
- Net Carbs: 0.6g
- Carbohydrate: 0.7g
- Fiber: 0.1g
- Protein: 61.5g
- Fat: 25.9g
- Sugar: 0g
- Sodium: 199mg

# Beef Taco Bake

**(Yields:** 6 servings / **Prep Time:** 15 minutes / **Cooking Time:** 1 hour**)**

## Ingredients

**For Crust:**
- 3 organic eggs
- 4 ounces cream cheese, softened
- ½ teaspoon taco seasoning
- 1/3 cup heavy cream
- 8 ounces cheddar cheese, shredded

**For Topping:**
- 1 pound grass-fed ground beef
- 4 ounces canned chopped green chilies
- ¼ cup sugar-free tomato sauce
- 3 teaspoons taco seasoning
- 8 ounces cheddar cheese, shredded

## Instructions

1. Preheat the oven to 375 degrees F. Lightly grease a 13x9-inch baking dish.
2. For crust: in a bowl, add the eggs, and cream cheese and beat until well combined and smooth.
3. Add the taco seasoning, and heavy cream and mix well.
4. Place cheddar cheese evenly in the bottom of prepared baking dish.
5. Spread cream cheese mixture evenly over cheese.
6. Bake for about 25-30 minutes.
7. Remove from the oven and set aside for about 5 minutes.
8. Meanwhile, for the topping: heat a large nonstick skillet over medium-high heat and cook the beef for about 8-10 minutes.
9. Drain the excess grease from skillet.
10. Stir in the green chilies, tomato sauce, and taco seasoning and remove from the heat.
11. Place the beef mixture evenly over crust and sprinkle with cheese.
12. Bake for about 18-20 minutes or until bubbly.
13. Remove from the oven and set aside for about 5 minutes.
14. Cut into desired size slices and serve.

## Nutrition Values (Per Serving)

- Calories: 569
- Net Carbs: 3.8g
- Carbohydrate: 4g
- Fiber: 0.2g
- Protein: 38.7g
- Fat: 43.7g
- Sugar: 1.8g
- Sodium: 773mg

---

# Beef Casserole

(**Yields:** 5 servings / **Prep Time:** 20 minutes / **Cooking Time:** 30 minutes)

## Ingredients

- 1 pound grass-fed ground beef
- 1 cup fresh mushrooms, sliced
- 2 celery stalks, chopped
- 1 small yellow onion, chopped

- 1 (12-ounces) bag French cut green beans
- 1 cup cheddar cheese, shredded
- ½ cup heavy cream
- 1/8 teaspoon garlic powder
- Salt and ground black pepper, as required

## Instructions

1. Preheat the oven to 350 degrees F. Lightly, grease a casserole dish
2. Heat a large nonstick skillet over medium-high heat and cook the beef, mushrooms, celery, and onion for about 6-7 minutes.
3. Remove the grease from skillet and set aside.
4. Meanwhile, arrange a steamer basket into a large pan of boiling water.
5. Place the green beans into steamer basket and steam, covered for about 4-5 minutes.
6. Remove from the pan and transfer green beans into a bowl.
7. For the sauce: in a microwave-safe bowl, add the cheddar, cream, garlic powder, salt, and black pepper and microwave for about 2-3 minutes, stirring frequently.
8. Place beef mixture and sauce into the prepared casserole dish and stir to combine well.
9. Bake for about 18-20 minutes or until bubbly.
10. Remove from the oven and set aside for about 5 minutes.
11. Cut into desired size slices and serve.

## Nutrition Values (Per Serving)

- Calories: 325
- Net Carbs: 5g
- Carbohydrate: 7.1g
- Fiber: 2.1g
- Protein: 26.5g
- Fat: 20.8g
- Sugar: 2.5g
- Sodium: 445mg

**(Tip:** If you are using a frozen beef, then make sure to thaw it before cooking.)

# Shepherd Pie

**(Yields:** 6 servings / **Prep Time:** 15 minutes / **Cooking Time:** 50 minutes)

## Ingredients

- 2 tablespoons olive oil
- 1 pound grass-fed ground beef
- ½ cup celery, chopped
- ¼ cup yellow onion, chopped
- 3 garlic cloves, minced
- 1 cup tomatoes, chopped
- 2 (12-ounces) packages riced cauliflower, cooked and well drained
- 1 cup cheddar cheese, shredded
- ¼ cup Parmesan cheese, shredded
- 1 cup heavy cream
- 1 teaspoon dried thyme

### Instructions

1. Preheat the oven to 350 degrees F.
2. Heat the oil in a large skillet over medium heat and cook the ground beef, celery, onions and garlic for about 8-10 minutes.
3. Remove from heat and drain the excess grease.
4. Immediately, stir in the tomatoes.
5. Transfer the mixture into a 10x7-inch casserole dish.
6. In a food processor, add the cauliflower, cheeses, cream, and thyme and pulse until mashed potatoes alike mixture is formed.
7. Spread the cauliflower mixture evenly over meat in the casserole dish.
8. Bake for about 35-40 minutes.
9. Remove from the oven and set aside to cool slightly before serving.
10. Cut into desired size pieces and serve.

### Nutrition Values (Per Serving)

- Calories: 411
- Net Carbs: 5.5g
- Carbohydrate: 9g
- Fiber: 3.5g
- Protein: 32g
- Fat: 27.9g
- Sugar: 4g
- Sodium: 274mg

===

## Beef Crust Pizza

**(Yields:** 8 servings / **Prep Time:** 15 minutes / **Cooking Time:** 23 minutes)

### Ingredients

- 2 pounds grass-fed lean ground beef
- ½ cup Parmesan cheese, grated
- 2 organic eggs
- 2 teaspoons Italian seasoning
- 1 teaspoon garlic powder
- Salt and ground black pepper, as required
- 9 ounces cooked spinach, chopped
- 2 tomatoes, sliced
- 2 cups mozzarella cheese, shredded

### Instructions

1. Preheat the oven to 450 degrees F.
2. In a bowl, add the beef, parmesan cheese, eggs, Italian seasoning, garlic powder, salt, and black pepper and mix until well combined.
3. Place the beef mixture onto a large baking sheet in a circle with slight sides.
4. Bake for about 20 minutes.
5. Remove from oven and carefully, discard the excess grease from baking sheet.
6. Arrange spinach and tomato slices on top of the beef crust and sprinkle with mozzarella cheese.

7. Now, set the oven to broiler on high.
8. Broil for about 2-3 minutes.
9. Cut into 8 equal-sized wedges and serve.

## **Nutrition Values (Per Serving)**

- Calories: 252
- Net Carbs: 2g
- Carbohydrate: 3.1g
- Fiber: 1.1g
- Protein: 27.8g
- Fat: 12.9g
- Sugar: 1.2g
- Sodium: 179mg

## **Beef Stuffed Bell Peppers**

**(Yields:** 6 servings **/ Prep Time:** 15 minutes **/ Cooking Time:** 20 minutes**)**

## **Ingredients**

- 1 pound grass-fed ground beef
- 1 garlic clove, minced
- 2 teaspoons coconut oil
- 1 cup white mushrooms, chopped
- 1 cup yellow onion, chopped
- 1 tablespoon red chili powder
- 1 tablespoon ground cumin
- ¼ teaspoon ground cinnamon
- Salt, as required
- ½ cup homemade tomato puree
- 3 large bell peppers, halved lengthwise and cored
- 1 cup water
- 4 ounces sharp cheddar cheese, shredded

## **Instructions**

1. Heat the oil in a skillet over medium-high heat and sauté the garlic for about 30 seconds.
2. Add the beef and cook for about 5 minutes, crumbling with the spoon
3. Add the mushrooms and onion and cook for about 5-6 minutes.
4. Stir in spices and cook for about 30 seconds.
5. Remove from the heat and stir in tomato puree.
6. Meanwhile, in a microwave-safe dish, arrange the bell peppers, cut-side down.
7. Pour the water in baking dish.
8. With a plastic wrap, cover the baking dish and microwave on high for about 4-5 minutes.
9. Remove from microwave and uncover the baking dish.
10. Dain the water completely
11. Now in the baking dish, arrange the bell peppers, cut-side up.
12. Stuff the bell peppers evenly with beef mixture and top with cheese.
13. Microwave on high for about 2-3 minutes.
14. Serve warm.

## Nutrition Values (Per Serving)

- Calories: 275
- Net Carbs: 7.6g
- Carbohydrate: 10g
- Fiber: 2.4g
- Protein: 29.5g
- Fat: 13.2g
- Sugar: 5.2g
- Sodium: 219mg

---

# Beef & Zucchini Lasagna

**(Yields:** 5 servings / **Prep Time:** 15 minutes / **Cooking Time:** 43 minutes)

## Ingredients

- 1 large zucchini
- Salt, to taste
- 1 pound grass-fed ground beef
- 1 cup sugar-free marinara sauce
- Ground black pepper, as required
- 10 ounces ricotta cheese
- 4 ounces mozzarella cheese, shredded

## Instructions

1. With a vegetable peeler, peel the zucchini into strips, leaving the core.
2. Sprinkle the zucchini strips with salt and set aside in a colander for about 15 minutes.
3. Carefully, squeeze out the zucchini strips to remove moisture.
4. Preheat the oven to 350 degrees F.
5. Heat a nonstick skillet and cook the ground beef for about 8-10 minutes.
6. Stir in the marinara sauce, salt, and black pepper and remove from heat.
7. In a casserole dish, evenly place the beef, followed by zucchini, ricotta and mozzarella.
8. With a piece of foil, cover the casserole dish and bake for about 30 minutes.
9. Now, set the oven to broiler.
10. Remove the foil and broil for about 2-3 minutes.
11. Cut into desired size pieces and serve.

## Nutrition Values (Per Serving)

- Calories: 153
- Net Carbs: 5.2g
- Carbohydrate: 5.9g
- Fiber: 0.7g
- Protein: 13.6g
- Fat: 8.6g
- Sugar: 1.3g
- Sodium: 244mg

# Beef Burgers with Yogurt Sauce

**(Yields:** 6 servings / **Prep Time:** 20 minutes / **Total Cooking Time:** 16 minutes)

## Ingredients

- 1 pound grass-fed ground beef
- 1 medium beetroot, trimmed, peeled and finely chopped
- 1 carrot, peeled and finely chopped
- 1 small yellow onion, finely chopped
- 1 tablespoon fresh rosemary, finely chopped
- Salt and ground black pepper, as required
- 2 tablespoons olive oil

**For Yogurt Sauce:**

- ¾ cup plain Greek yogurt
- 1 teaspoon fresh lemon juice
- 1 teaspoon garlic, minced
- 1 teaspoon fresh oregano, chopped
- Salt, as required
- ½ teaspoon granulated Erythritol

## Instructions

1. For burgers: in a large bowl, add the beef, veggies, rosemary, salt, and black pepper and mix until well combined.
2. Make 12 equal-sized patties from the mixture.
3. Heat the oil in a large skillet over medium heat and cook the patties in 2 batches for about 3-4 minutes per side or until golden brown.
4. Meanwhile, for the yogurt sauce: place all the ingredients in a serving bowl and mix until well combined.
5. Divide two patties onto each serving plate and serve alongside the yogurt sauce.

## Nutrition Values (Per Serving)

- Calories: 229
- Net Carbs: 6.1g
- Carbohydrate: 7.3g
- Fiber: 1.2g
- Protein: 25.8g
- Fat: 3.10g
- Sugar: 5.2g
- Sodium: 293mg

---

# Lamb Stew

**(Yields:** 8 servings / **Prep Time:** 15 minutes / **Cooking Time:** 2¼ hours)

## Ingredients

- 1 teaspoon ground coriander
- ¾ teaspoon ground cumin
- ½ teaspoon cayenne pepper
- 2 tablespoons coconut oil
- 3 pounds grass-fed lamb stew meat, cubed

- Salt and ground black pepper, as required
- ½ yellow onion, chopped
- 2 garlic cloves, minced
- 2 cups homemade chicken broth
- 1 (15-ounces) can sugar-free diced tomatoes
- 1 medium head cauliflower, cut into 1-inch florets

## Instructions

1. Preheat the oven to 300 degrees F.
2. In a small bowl, mix together the spices and set aside.
3. In a large ovenproof pan, heat the oil over medium heat and cook the lamb with salt and black pepper for about 10 minutes or until browned from all sides.
4. With a slotted spoon, transfer the lamb into a bowl.
5. In the same pan, add onion and sauté for about 3-4 minutes.
6. Add the garlic and spice mixture and sauté for about 1 minute.
7. Add the cooked lamb, broth, and tomatoes and bring to a gentle boil.
8. Immediately, cover the pan with lid and transfer into oven.
9. Bake for about 1½ hours.
10. Remove from oven and stir in the cauliflower.
11. Bake, covered for about 30 more minutes or until cauliflower is done completely.
12. Serve hot.

## Nutrition Values (Per Serving)

- Calories: 379
- Net Carbs: 3.4g
- Carbohydrate: 5.2g
- Fiber: 1.8g
- Protein: 50.3g
- Fat: 16.4g
- Sugar: 2.7g
- Sodium: 353mg

# Lamb Curry

(**Yields:** 4 servings / **Prep Time:** 15 minutes / **Cooking Time:** 1 hour 50 minutes)

## Ingredients

- 1 tablespoon olive oil
- 1 pound grass-fed boneless lamb, cubed
- 1 celery stalk, chopped
- 1 small yellow onion, chopped
- 1/3 of fresh red chili, chopped
- 1 teaspoon butter
- 2 garlic cloves, minced
- 2 teaspoons garam masala powder
- 1 teaspoon red chili powder
- ¼ teaspoon ground turmeric
- 1 tablespoon sugar-free tomato paste
- 1 cup unsweetened coconut milk
- ½ cup water

- 1 medium carrot, peeled and chopped
- 1 teaspoon fresh lime juice
- Salt and ground black pepper, as required
- 2 tablespoons fresh cilantro leaves, chopped

## Instructions

1. In a large pan, heat the oil over high heat and sear the lamb cubes for about 4-5 minutes.
2. Add the onion, celery, and red chili and cook for about 1 minute.
3. Now, adjust the heat to medium.
4. Stir in the butter, garlic, and spices and cook for about 1 minute.
5. Stir in the tomato paste, coconut milk, and water and bring to a boil.
6. Adjust the heat to low and simmer, covered for about 1 hour, stirring occasionally.
7. Stir in the carrot and simmer, covered for about 40 minutes.
8. Stir in the lime juice, salt, and black pepper and remove from heat.
9. Garnish with fresh cilantro and serve hot.

## Nutrition Values (Per Serving)

- Calories: 410
- Net Carbs: 5.8g
- Carbohydrate: 8.4g
- Fiber: 2.6g
- Protein: 34g
- Fat: 27.3g
- Sugar: 4.1g
- Sodium: 169mg

---

# Lamb with Cabbage

**(Yields:** 5 servings / **Prep Time:** 15 minutes / **Cooking Time:** 20 minutes)

## Ingredients

- 4 bacon slices, chopped
- 1 pound grass-fed ground lamb
- ¼ cup green bell pepper, seeded and chopped
- ¼ cup yellow onion, chopped
- 1 teaspoon garlic, minced
- 4 cups green cabbage, thinly sliced
- 1 (15-ounces) can sugar-free tomato sauce
- Salt and ground black pepper, as required

## Instructions

1. Heat a large nonstick skillet over medium heat and cook the bacon for about 5 minutes, stirring occasionally.
2. Add the ground lamb, bell pepper, onion, and garlic and cook for about 7-8 minutes, stirring occasionally.

3. Stir in the cabbage, and tomato sauce and cook, covered for about 5-7 minutes or until desired doneness.
4. Stir in the salt, and black pepper and remove from the heat.
5. Serve hot.

## Nutrition Values (Per Serving)

- Calories: 333
- Net Carbs: 7.1g
- Carbohydrate: 9.2g
- Fiber: 2.1g
- Protein: 36.1g
- Fat: 16.6g
- Sugar: 5.4g
- Sodium: 1200mg

# Grilled Lamb Burgers

(**Yields:** 4 servings / **Prep Time:** 15 minutes / **Total Cooking Time:** 8 minutes)

## Ingredients

- 1 pound grass-fed ground lamb
- ¼ yellow onion, chopped
- 2 garlic cloves, minced
- 2 teaspoons fresh oregano, minced
- 1 teaspoon fresh lemon zest, finely grated
- Salt and ground black pepper, as required
- 6 cups lettuce

## Instructions

1. Preheat the grill to medium-high heat. Grease the grill grate.
2. In a bowl, add the lamb, onion, garlic, oregano, lemon zest, salt, and black pepper and with your hands, mix until well combined.
3. Make 8 small equal-sized patties from the mixture.
4. Grill the patties for about 4 minutes per side or until desired doneness.
5. Divide the lettuces onto serving plates.
6. Top each with 2 burgers and serve.

## Nutrition Values (Per Serving)

- Calories: 230
- Net Carbs: 3.3g
- Carbohydrate: 4.4g
- Fiber: 1.1g
- Protein: 32.5g
- Fat: 8.6g
- Sugar: 1.2g
- Sodium: 325mg

(**Tip:** Make sure the grill is heated to appropriate temperature before cooking the burgers.)

# Roasted Lamb Shanks

**(Yields:** 4 servings / **Prep Time:** 15 minutes / **Cooking Time:** 3 hours 5 minutes)

## Ingredients

- 2 teaspoons ground cumin
- 2 teaspoons onion powder
- ½ teaspoon cayenne pepper
- Salt and ground black pepper, as required
- 4 (12-14 ounces) grass-fed lamb shanks, rinsed and dried
- 10 garlic cloves, peeled
- ½ cup olive oil, divided
- 3 teaspoons dried oregano, crushed
- ½ cup fresh lemon juice
- 1 cup water

## Instructions

1. Preheat the oven to 450 degrees F. Grease a large roasting pan.
2. In a small bowl, mix well cumin, onion powder, cayenne pepper, salt, and black pepper.
3. Coat the lamb shanks evenly with spice mixture.
4. In the bottom of prepared roasting pan, evenly spread the garlic cloves.
5. Arrange the lamb shanks on top of garlic and drizzle with 2 tablespoons of oil.
6. Roast for about 35 minutes.
7. Remove the roasting pan from oven.
8. Now, adjust the temperature of oven to 350 degrees F.
9. In a bowl, add the remaining oil, oregano, lemon juice, and water and mix until well combined.
10. Place the oil mixture evenly over lamb shanks.
11. With a piece of foil, cover the roasting pan and roast for about 2½ hours.
12. Remove from the oven and serve hot.

## Nutrition Values (Per Serving)

- Calories: 879
- Net Carbs: 4.4g
- Carbohydrate: 5.3g
- Fiber: 0.9g
- Protein: 96.7g
- Fat: 50.g
- Sugar: 1.2g
- Sodium: 307mg

---

# Lamb Chops with Garlic Sauce

**(Yields:** 4 servings / **Prep Time:** 15 minutes / **Cooking Time:** 8 minutes)

## Ingredients

- 3 tablespoons butter
- 10 small garlic cloves, halved

- 8 (4-ounces) (½-inch thick) grass-fed lamb loin chops, trimmed
- ¼ teaspoon dried thyme, crushed
- ¼ teaspoon red pepper flakes, crushed
- Salt and ground black pepper, as required
- 2 tablespoons fresh lemon juice
- 3 tablespoons water
- 3 tablespoons fresh parsley, finely chopped and divided

## Instructions

1. Heat the butter in a large skillet over medium-high and sauté garlic for about 1 minute.
2. Add the lamb chops, thyme, red pepper flakes, salt, and black pepper and cook for about 3-4 minutes.
3. Flip the side and cook for about 2-3 more minutes.
4. Divide the chops onto serving plates, leaving the garlic in skillet.
5. In the skillet, add the lemon juice, water and half of the parsley and cook for about 1 minute, stirring continuously.
6. Pour the sauce evenly over chops.
7. Garnish with the remaining parsley and serve.

## Nutrition Values (Per Serving)

- Calories: 513
- Net Carbs: 2.6g
- Carbohydrate: 2.9g
- Fiber: 0.3g
- Protein: 64.4g
- Fat: 25.4g
- Sugar: 0.3g
- Sodium: 277mg

(**Tip:** For the best result, avoid the over-cooking of lamb chops.)

## Lamb Chops with Cream Sauce

(**Yields:** 3 servings / **Prep Time:** 14 minutes / **Cooking Time:** 30 minutes)

## Ingredients

- 1½ pounds grass-fed lamb chops, trimmed
- 2 garlic cloves, minced
- 1 tablespoon fresh rosemary, minced
- 2 tablespoons olive oil, divided
- Salt and ground black pepper, as required
- 1 tablespoon yellow onion, minced
- ½ cup homemade chicken broth
- 3 tablespoons fresh lemon juice
- 2/3 cup heavy cream
- 1 tablespoon mustard
- 2 teaspoons Worcestershire sauce
- 1 teaspoon Erythritol
- 1 fresh thyme sprig
- 1 fresh rosemary sprig
- 2 tablespoons butter

## Instructions

1. In a shallow baking dish, mix well garlic, rosemary, 1 tablespoon of oil, salt and black pepper.
2. Add the lamb chops and evenly coat with oil mixture.
3. Now, arrange the lamb chops in a single layer.
4. With a plastic wrap, cover the baking dish and refrigerate overnight.
5. Remove from refrigerator and place the lamb chops at room temperature for about 30 minutes before cooking.
6. Heat the remaining oil in a large nonstick skillet over medium heat.
7. Place the lamb chops in a single layer and cook for about 6-7 minutes per side.
8. With a slotted spoon, transfer the lamb chops onto a plate and loosely cover with a piece of foil to keep warm.
9. In the same skillet, add the onion over medium-low heat and sauté for about 2-3 minutes.
10. Add the broth and lemon juice and bring to a boil.
11. Cook for about 1 minute.
12. Add the Worcestershire sauce, mustard, and Erythritol and stir to combine well.
13. Stir in the cream, and herb sprigs and cook for about 7-8 minutes, stirring frequently.
14. Stir in the butter and cook for about 1-2 minutes, stirring frequently.
15. Remove the skillet of sauce from heat and discard the herb sprigs.
16. Place the sauce over lamb chops and serve.

## Nutrition Values (Per Serving)

- Calories: 704
- Net Carbs: 3.9g
- Carbohydrate: 5.6g
- Fiber: 1.7g
- Protein: 66.5g
- Fat: 45.3g
- Sugar: 1.6g
- Sodium: 406mg

---

# Grilled Rack of Lamb

**(Yields:** 8 servings / **Prep Time:** 15 minutes / **Cooking Time:** 29 minutes)

## Ingredients

- 2 (2½-pounds) grass-fed racks of lamb, chine bones removed and trimmed
- Salt and ground black pepper, as required
- 2 tablespoons Dijon mustard
- 2 teaspoons rosemary, chopped
- 2 teaspoons fresh parsley, chopped
- 2 teaspoons fresh thyme, chopped

## Instructions

1. Preheat the charcoal grill to high heat. Grease the grill grate.
2. Season the rack of lamb evenly with salt and black pepper.
3. Coat the meaty sides of racks with mustard, followed by fresh herbs, pressing gently.
4. Push the coals to one side of grill.
5. Place racks of lamb over the coals, meaty side down and cook for about 6 minutes.
6. Flip and cook for about 3 more minutes.
7. Again, flip the racks down and move racks to the cooler side of grill.
8. Cover the grill and cook for about 20 minutes.
9. Remove from the grill and place racks of lamb onto a cutting board for about 10 minutes.
10. With a sharp knife, carve the racks of lamb into chops and serve.

## Nutrition Values (Per Serving)

- Calories: 532
- Net Carbs: 0.2g
- Carbohydrate: 0.6g
- Fiber: 0.4g
- Protein: 79.8g
- Fat: 21g
- Sugar: 0g
- Sodium: 260mg

---

# Broiled Lamb Chops

**(Yields:** 4 servings / **Prep Time:** 15 minutes / **Total Cooking Time:** 8 minutes)

## Ingredients

- 2 tablespoons garlic, minced
- 2 tablespoons fresh oregano, minced
- ½ teaspoon fresh lemon zest, finely grated
- 1 tablespoon olive oil
- 2 tablespoons fresh lemon juice
- Salt and ground black pepper, as required
- 8 (4-ounces) grass-fed lamb loin chops, trimmed
- 2 tablespoons Parmesan cheese, shredded

## Instructions

1. Place all the ingredients except lamb chops and Parmesan in a large baking dish and mix until well combined.
2. Add the chops and generously coat with garlic mixture.

3. Cover the baking dish and refrigerate to marinate for at least 1 hour.
4. Preheat the broiler of oven to high heat. Grease a broiler pan.
5. Arrange the chops onto prepared broiler pan in a single layer.
6. Broil for about 3-4 minutes per side.
7. Sprinkle with Parmesan cheese and serve hot.

## Nutrition Values (Per Serving)

- Calories: 477
- Net Carbs: 2g
- Carbohydrate: 3.1g
- Fiber: 1.1g
- Protein: 65.2g
- Fat: 21.1g
- Sugar: 0.3g
- Sodium: 256mg

---

## Baked Lamb Chops

(**Yields:** 4 servings / **Prep Time:** 15 minutes / **Total Cooking Time:** 16 minutes)

## Ingredients

- ¼ cup olive oil
- 2 garlic cloves, crushed
- 1 teaspoon fresh lemon zest, finely grated
- 1 teaspoon dried oregano, crushed
- Salt and ground black pepper, as required
- 8 (4-ounces) grass-fed lamb loin chops, trimmed

## Instructions

1. In a large glass dish, mix well oil, garlic, lemon zest, oregano, salt and black pepper.
2. Add the lamb chops and generously coat with oil mixture.
3. Refrigerate to marinate for about 4 hours.
4. Preheat the oven to 400 degrees F.
5. Remove the lamb chops from bowl and shake to remove any marinade.
6. Heat a large ovenproof skillet over medium-high heat and sear the chops for about 3 minutes per side.
7. Transfer the skillet into oven and roast for about 8-10 minutes.
8. Remove from the oven and set aside for about 2 minutes before serving.

## Nutrition Values (Per Serving)

- Calories: 534
- Net Carbs: 0.6g
- Carbohydrate: 0.8g
- Fiber: 0.2g
- Protein: 63.9g
- Fat: 29.3g
- Sugar: 0.1g
- Sodium: 554mg

## Grilled Leg of Lamb

**(Yields:** 10 servings / **Prep Time:** 15 minutes / **Cooking Time:** 30 minutes)

## Ingredients

- 1/3 cup olive oil
- ¼ cup fresh lemon juice
- 6 garlic cloves, chopped
- ½ cup fresh oregano, chopped
- Salt and ground black pepper, as required
- 1 (4½-pounds) grass-fed boneless leg of lamb, trimmed and butterflied

## Instructions

1. In a shallow glass baking dish, mix well oil, lemon juice, garlic, oregano, salt, and black pepper.
2. Add the leg of lamb and generously coat with the mixture.
3. Cover the baking dish and refrigerate to marinate overnight, flipping occasionally.
4. Preheat the charcoal grill to medium-high heat. Grease the grill grate.
5. Remove the leg of lamb from refrigerator.
6. Carefully, insert a long metal skewer crosswise in the butterflied leg.
7. Place leg of lamb onto the grill and cook for about 20-30 minutes, flipping occasionally.
8. Remove from oven and place the leg of lamb over a cutting board.
9. With a piece of foil, cover the leg loosely for about 5-10 minutes before slicing.
10. With a sharp knife, cut the leg of lamb into desired size slices and serve.

## Nutrition Values (Per Serving)

- Calories: 452
- Net Carbs: 1.5g
- Carbohydrate: 3.1g
- Fiber: 1.6g
- Protein: 57.9g
- Fat: 22.1g
- Sugar: 0.3g
- Sodium: 173mg

---

## Roasted Leg of Lamb

**(Yields:** 8 servings / **Prep Time:** 15 minutes / **Cooking Time:** 1½ hours)

## Ingredients

- 1/3 cup fresh parsley, minced
- 4 garlic cloves, minced

- 1 teaspoon fresh lemon zest, finely grated
- 1 tablespoon ground coriander
- 1 tablespoon ground cumin
- 1 tablespoon smoked paprika
- 1 tablespoon red pepper flakes, finely crushed
- ½ teaspoon ground allspice
- 1/3 cup olive oil
- 1 (5-pounds) grass-fed bone-in leg of lamb, trimmed

## **Instructions**

1. Add all the ingredients in a mixing bowl except leg of lamb and mix well.
2. Generously coat the leg of lamb with marinade mixture.
3. With a plastic wrap, cover the leg of lamb and refrigerate to marinate for about 6-8 hours.
4. Remove from refrigerator and keep in room temperature for about 30 minutes before roasting.
5. Preheat the oven to 350 degrees F. Arrange the oven rack in the center of oven.
6. Arrange a lightly, greased rack in the roasting pan.
7. Place the leg of lamb over rack into the roasting pan.
8. Roast for about 1¼-1½ hours, rotating the pan once halfway through.
9. Remove from oven and place the leg of lamb onto a cutting board for about 10-15 minutes.
10. With a sharp knife, cut the leg of lamb into desired size slices and serve.

## **Nutrition Values (Per Serving)**

- Calories: 610
- Net Carbs: 1.3g
- Carbohydrate: 2g
- Fiber: 0.7g
- Protein: 80.1g
- Fat: 29.6g
- Sugar: 0.2g
- Sodium: 219mg

---

## **Stuffed Leg of Lamb**

(**Yields:** 10 servings / **Prep Time:** 15 minutes / **Cooking Time:** 1 hour 40 minutes)

## **Ingredients**

- 1/3 cup fresh parsley, minced
- 8 garlic cloves, minced and divided
- 3 tablespoons olive oil, divided
- Salt and ground black pepper, as required

- 1 (4-pounds) grass-fed boneless leg of lamb, butterflied and trimmed
- 1/3 cup yellow onion, minced
- 1 bunch fresh kale, trimmed and chopped
- ½ cup Kalamata olives, pitted and chopped
- ½ cup feta cheese, crumbled
- 1 teaspoon fresh lemon zest, finely grated

## **Instructions**

1. In a large baking dish, add the parsley, 4 garlic cloves, 2 tablespoons of oil, salt, and black pepper and mix until well combined.
2. Add the leg of lamb and generously coat with parsley mixture. Set aside at room temperature.
3. In a large skillet, heat the remaining oil over medium heat and sauté the onion and remaining garlic for about 4-5 minutes.
4. Add the kale and cook for about 4-5 minutes.
5. Remove from the heat and set aside to cool for at least 10 minutes.
6. Stir in the remaining ingredients.
7. Preheat the oven to 450 degrees F. Grease a shallow roasting pan.
8. Place the leg of lamb onto a smooth surface, cut-side up.
9. Place kale mixture in the center, leaving 1-inch border from both sides.
10. Roll the short side to seal the stuffing and with a kitchen string, tightly tie the roll at many places.
11. Arrange the roll into prepared roasting pan, seam-side down.
12. Roast for about 15 minutes.
13. Now, adjust the temperature of oven to 350 degrees F.
14. Roast for about 1-1¼ hours.
15. Remove the leg of lamb from oven and place onto a cutting board for about 10-20 minutes before slicing.
16. With a sharp knife, cut the roll into desired size slices and serve.

## **Nutrition Values (Per Serving)**

- Calories: 346
- Net Carbs: 2.4g
- Carbohydrate: 2.9g
- Fiber: 0.5g
- Protein: 44g
- Fat: 16.5g
- Sugar: 0.4g
- Sodium: 251mg

# CHAPTER 4 | PORK

## Meatballs Curry

**(Yields:** 6 servings / **Prep Time:** 15 minutes / **Cooking Time:** 25 minutes)

## Ingredients

**For Meatballs:**

- 1 pound lean ground pork
- 2 organic eggs, beaten
- 3 tablespoons yellow onion, finely chopped
- ¼ cup fresh parsley leaves, chopped
- ¼ teaspoon fresh ginger, minced
- 2 garlic cloves, minced
- 1 jalapeño pepper, seeded and finely chopped
- 1 teaspoon Erythritol
- 1 tablespoon red curry paste
- 3 tablespoons olive oil

**For Curry:**

- 1 yellow onion, chopped
- Salt, as required
- 2 garlic cloves, minced
- ¼ teaspoon fresh ginger, minced
- 2 tablespoons red curry paste
- 1 (14-ounces) can unsweetened coconut milk
- Ground black pepper, as required
- ¼ cup fresh parsley, chopped

## Instructions

1. For meatballs: place all the ingredients except oil in a large bowl and mix until well combined.
2. Make small-sized balls from the mixture.
3. Heat the oil in a large wok over medium heat and cook meatballs for about 3-5 minutes or until golden brown from all sides.
4. Transfer the meatballs into a bowl.
5. For curry: in the same wok, add onion, and a pinch of salt and sauté for about 4-5 minutes.
6. Add the garlic, and ginger and sauté for about 1 minute.
7. Add the curry paste, and sauté for about 1-2 minutes.
8. Add coconut milk, and meatballs and bring to a gentle simmer.
9. Adjust the heat to low and simmer, covered for about 10-12 minutes.
10. Season with salt and black pepper and remove from the heat.
11. Top with fresh parsley and serve.

## Nutrition Values (Per Serving)

- Calories: 444
- Net Carbs: 6.4g
- Carbohydrate: 8.6g
- Fiber: 2.2g
- Protein: 17g
- Fat: 39.3g
- Sugar: 3.3g
- Sodium: 192mg

# Meatballs in Cheese Sauce

**(Yields:** 5 servings / **Prep Time:** 20 minutes / **Cooking Time:** 25 minutes)

## Ingredients

### For Meatballs:

- 1 pound ground pork
- 1 organic egg, beaten
- 2 ounces Parmesan cheese, grated
- ½ tablespoon dried basil
- 1 teaspoon garlic powder
- ½ teaspoon onion powder
- Salt and ground black pepper, as required
- 3 tablespoons olive oil

### For Sauce:

- 1 (14-ounces) can sugar-free diced tomatoes
- 2 tablespoons butter
- 7 ounces fresh spinach
- 2 tablespoons fresh parsley, chopped
- 5 ounces mozzarella cheese, grated
- Salt and ground black pepper, as required

## Instructions

1. For meatballs: add all the ingredients except oil in a large bowl and mix until well combined.
2. Make small-sized balls from the mixture.
3. Heat the oil in a large wok over medium heat and cook the meatballs for about 3-5 minutes or until golden brown from all sides.
4. Add the tomatoes and stir to combine.
5. Adjust the heat to low and simmer for about 15 minutes, stirring occasionally.
6. Meanwhile, melt the butter in another wok over medium heat and stir fry the spinach for about 1-2 minutes.
7. Season with salt, and black pepper and remove from the heat.
8. Add the cooked spinach, parsley and mozzarella cheese into the wok of meatballs and stir to combine.
9. Cook for about 1-2 minutes.
10. Remove from the heat and serve.

## Nutrition Values (Per Serving)

- Calories: 398
- Net Carbs: 4.7g
- Carbohydrate: 6.6g
- Fiber: 1.9g
- Protein: 38.6g
- Fat: 24.8g
- Sugar: 2.6g
- Sodium: 439mg

# Chocolate Chili

**(Yields:** 8 servings / **Prep Time:** 15 minutes / **Cooking Time:** 2¼ hours)

## Ingredients

- 2 tablespoons olive oil
- 1 small onion, chopped
- 1 green bell pepper, seeded and chopped
- 4 garlic cloves, minced
- 1 jalapeño pepper, chopped
- 1 teaspoon dried thyme, crushed
- 2 tablespoons red chili powder
- 1 tablespoon ground cumin
- 2 pounds lean ground pork
- 2 cups fresh tomatoes, finely chopped
- 4 ounces sugar-free tomato paste
- 1½ tablespoons cacao powder
- 2 cups chicken broth
- 1 cup water
- Salt and ground black pepper, as required
- ¼ cup cheddar cheese, shredded

## Instructions

1. Heat the oil in a large pan over medium heat and sauté the onion and bell pepper for about 5-7 minutes.
2. Add the garlic, jalapeño pepper, thyme, and spices and sauté for about 1 minute.
3. Add the pork and cook for about 4-5 minutes.
4. Stir in the tomatoes, tomato paste, and cacao powder and cook for about 2 minutes.
5. Add the broth, and water and bring to a boil.
6. Adjust the heat to low and simmer, covered for about 2 hours.
7. Stir in the salt, and black pepper and remove from heat.
8. Top with cheddar cheese and serve hot.

## Nutrition Values (Per Serving)

- Calories: 326
- Net Carbs: 6.5g
- Carbohydrate: 9.1g
- Fiber: 2.6g
- Protein: 23.3g
- Fat: 22.9g
- Sugar: 4.5g
- Sodium: 270mg

---

# Pork Stew

**(Yields:** 6 servings / **Prep Time:** 15 minutes / **Cooking Time:** 45 minutes)

## Ingredients

- 2 tablespoons olive oil
- 2 teaspoons paprika

- 2 pounds pork tenderloin, cut into 1-inch cubes
- 1 tablespoon garlic, minced
- ¾ cup homemade chicken broth
- 1 cup sugar-free tomato sauce
- ½ tablespoon Erythritol
- 1 teaspoon dried oregano
- 2 dried bay leaves
- 2 tablespoons fresh lemon juice
- Salt and ground black pepper, as required

## Instructions

1. Heat the oil in a large heavy-bottomed pan over medium-high heat and cook the pork for about 3-4 minutes or until browned completely.
2. Add the garlic and cook for about 1 minute.
3. Stir in the remaining ingredients and bring to a boil.
4. Adjust the heat to medium-low and simmer, covered for about 30-40 minutes
5. Remove from heat and discard the bay leaves.
6. Serve hot.

## Nutrition Values (Per Serving)

- Calories: 277
- Net Carbs: 2.5g
- Carbohydrate: 3.6g
- Fiber: 1.1g
- Protein: 41g
- Fat: 10.4g
- Sugar: 2g
- Sodium: 785mg

## Pork & Chiles Stew

**(Yields:** 8 servings / **Prep Time:** 15 minutes / **Total Cooking Time:** 2 hrs. 10 mins)

## Ingredients

- 3 tablespoons unsalted butter
- 2½ pounds boneless pork ribs, cut into ¾-inch cubes
- 1 large yellow onion, chopped
- 4 garlic cloves, crushed
- 1½ cups homemade chicken broth
- 2 (10-ounces) cans sugar-free diced tomatoes
- 1 cup canned roasted poblano chiles
- 2 teaspoons dried oregano
- 1 teaspoon ground cumin
- Salt, as required
- ¼ cup fresh cilantro, chopped
- 2 tablespoons fresh lime juice

## Instructions

1. In a large pan, melt the butter over medium-high heat and cook the pork, onions and garlic for about 5 minutes or until browned.
2. Add the broth and scrape up the browned bits.

3. Add the tomatoes, poblano chiles, oregano, cumin, and salt and bring to a boil.
4. Adjust the heat to medium-low and simmer, covered for about 2 hours.
5. Stir in the fresh cilantro and lime juice and remove from heat.
6. Serve hot.

## Nutrition Values (Per Serving)

- Calories: 288
- Net Carbs: 6g
- Carbohydrate: 8.8g
- Fiber: 2.8g
- Protein: 39.6g
- Fat: 10.1g
- Sugar: 4g
- Sodium: 283mg

(**Note:** Poblano chiles can be replaced with Anaheim pepper.)

---

# Pork Stroganoff

(**Yields:** 5 servings / **Prep Time:** 15 minutes / **Total Cooking Time:** 40 minutes)

## Ingredients

- 1 pound pork loin, trimmed and cut into about 1-inch cubes
- 2 tablespoons Spanish paprika, divided
- Salt and ground black pepper, as required
- 3 tablespoons butter, divided
- 12 ounces fresh white mushrooms, cut into thick slices
- 1 yellow onion, finely chopped
- 1 teaspoon garlic, finely minced
- ½ teaspoon dried thyme
- 1 (14½-ounces) can petite diced tomatoes with juice
- ½ cup homemade chicken broth
- 2/3 cup heavy cream
- 1 tablespoon fresh lemon juice

## Instructions

1. In a bowl, add the pork cubes, 1 tablespoon of paprika, salt, and black pepper and toss to coat well.
2. In a heavy wok, melt 1 tablespoon of butter over medium-high heat and sear the pork cubes for about 5-6 minutes.
3. With a slotted spoon, transfer the pork cubes onto a plate.
4. In the same wok, melt 1 tablespoon of butter over medium heat and cook the mushrooms for about 5 minutes.
5. With a slotted spoon, transfer the mushrooms onto a plate.
6. In the same wok again, melt the remaining butter over medium heat and sauté the onion for about 3-5 minutes.
7. Add the garlic, thyme, and remaining paprika and sauté for about 1-2 minutes.

8. Add the tomatoes with juice, and broth and bring to a boil.
9. Cook for about 10 minutes or until the mixture becomes slightly thick.
10. Stir in the cooked pork cubes, and mushrooms and simmer, covered for about 10 minutes.
11. Remove the wok from heat and immediately, stir in the cream, lemon juice, salt, and black pepper.
12. Serve hot.

## **Nutrition Values (Per Serving)**

- Calories: 338
- Net Carbs: 6.6g
- Carbohydrate: 9.8g
- Fiber: 3.2g
- Protein: 29.2g
- Fat: 26.4g
- Sugar: 4g
- Sodium: 198mg

(**Note:** You can replace the heavy cream with sour cream if you desired.)

# Pork with Sauerkraut

(**Yields:** 8 servings / **Prep Time:** 15 minutes / **Cooking Time:** 2 hours 12 minutes)

## **Ingredients**

- 24 ounces sauerkraut
- 2 pounds pork roast
- Salt and ground black pepper, as required
- ¼ cup unsalted butter
- ½ yellow onion, thinly sliced
- 14 ounces precooked kielbasa, sliced into ½-inch rounds

## **Instructions**

1. Preheat the oven to 325 degrees F.
2. Drain the sauerkraut, reserving about 1 cup of liquid.
3. Lightly, season the pork roast with salt and black pepper.
4. Melt the butter in a heavy-bottomed wok over high heat and sear the pork for about 5-6 minutes per side.
5. With a slotted spoon, transfer the pork onto a plate.
6. In the bottom of a casserole, place half of sauerkraut and onion slices.
7. Add the seared pork roast and kielbasa pieces on top.
8. Top with the remaining sauerkraut and onion slices.
9. Add the reserved sauerkraut liquid into casserole dish.
10. Cover the casserole dish tightly and bake for about 2 hours.
11. Remove from oven and with tongs, transfer the pork roast onto a cutting board for at least 15 minutes.

12. With a sharp knife, cut the pork roast into desired size slices.
13. Divide the pork slices evenly onto serving plates and serve alongside the sauerkraut mixture.

## **Nutrition Values (Per Serving)**

- Calories: 417
- Net Carbs: 3.6g
- Carbohydrate: 6.3g
- Fiber: 2.7g
- Protein: 39.7g
- Fat: 25.3g
- Sugar: 1.8g
- Sodium: 1200mg

**(Tip:** Just before using, give sauerkraut a quick rinse.)

---

# **Fried Pork & Cilantro**

**(Yields:** 4 servings / **Prep Time:** 15 minutes / **Cooking Time:** 15 minutes)

## **Ingredients**

- 1 pound tender pork, trimmed and thinly sliced
- 1 tablespoon fresh ginger, finely chopped
- 4 garlic cloves, finely chopped
- 1 cup fresh cilantro, chopped and divided
- ¼ cup plus 1 tablespoon olive oil, divided
- 1 yellow onion, thinly sliced
- 1 large green bell pepper, seeded and thinly sliced
- 1 tablespoon fresh lime juice
- Salt and ground black pepper, as required

## **Instructions**

1. In a large bowl, mix well pork, ginger, garlic, ½ cup of cilantro and ¼ cup of oil.
2. Refrigerate to marinate for about 2 hours.
3. Heat a large wok over medium-high heat and stir fry the pork with marinade for about 4-5 minutes.
4. Transfer the pork into a bowl.
5. In the same wok, heat the remaining oil over medium heat and sauté the onion for about 3-4 minutes.
6. Stir in the bell pepper and stir fry for about 3-4 minutes.
7. Stir in the cooked pork, lime juice, remaining cilantro, salt, and black pepper and cook for about 2 minutes.
8. Remove from the heat and serve hot.

## Nutrition Values (Per Serving)

- Calories: 343
- Net Carbs: 5.6g
- Carbohydrate: 7g
- Fiber: 1.4g
- Protein: 30.7g
- Fat: 21.7g
- Sugar: 2.8g
- Sodium: 108mg

---

# Pork with Brussels Sprout

**(Yields:** 5 serving / **Prep Time:** 15 minutes / **Cooking Time:** 10 minutes)

## Ingredients

- 3 tablespoons butter
- 1 1/3 pounds pork belly, cut into bite-sized pieces
- 1 pound fresh Brussels sprouts, trimmed and halved
- 2 garlic cloves, minced
- 2 tablespoons low-sodium soy sauce
- 1 tablespoon balsamic vinegar
- Ground black pepper, as required
- 1 scallion, sliced

## Instructions

1. Melt the butter in a large wok over medium-high heat and cook the pork pieces for about 3-4 minutes or until golden brown.
2. Stir in the Brussels sprouts, and garlic and stir fry for about 3-4 minutes.
3. Add the soy sauce, vinegar, and black pepper and cook for about 1-2 minutes.
4. Stir in the scallion and serve hot.

## Nutrition Values (Per Serving)

- Calories: 348
- Net Carbs: 7.1g
- Carbohydrate: 11.6g
- Fiber: 4.5g
- Protein: 44.2g
- Fat: 14.4g
- Sugar: 3.1g
- Sodium: 617mg

# Pork with Veggies

**(Yields:** 4 servings / **Prep Time:** 15 minutes / **Cooking Time:** 10 minutes)

## Ingredients

- ¾ pound pork loin, cut into thin strips
- 2 tablespoons olive oil, divided
- 1 teaspoon garlic, minced
- 1 teaspoon fresh ginger, minced
- 2 tablespoons low-sodium soy sauce
- 1 tablespoon fresh lemon juice
- 1 teaspoon sesame oil
- 1 tablespoon Swerve
- 1 teaspoon arrowroot starch
- 12 ounces broccoli florets
- 1 large red bell pepper, seeded and cut into strips
- 2 scallions, cut into 2-inch pieces

## Instructions

1. In a bowl, mix well pork strips, ½ tablespoon of olive oil, garlic, and ginger.
2. For sauce; add the soy sauce, lemon juice, sesame oil, Swerve, and arrowroot starch in a small bowl and mix well.
3. Heat the remaining olive oil in a large nonstick wok over high heat and sear the pork strips for about 3-4 minutes or until cooked through.
4. With a slotted spoon, transfer the pork into a bowl.
5. In the same wok, add broccoli, bell pepper, and scallion and cook, covered for about 1-2 minutes.
6. Stir the cooked pork and sauce, and stir fry and cook for about 2-3 minutes or until desired doneness, stirring occasionally.
7. Remove from the heat and serve.

## Nutrition Values (Per Serving)

- Calories: 382
- Net Carbs: 7g
- Carbohydrate: 10g
- Fiber: 3g
- Protein: 34.4g
- Fat: 23.2g
- Sugar: 2.9g
- Sodium: 541mg

---

# Pork Liver with Scallion

**(Yields:** 3 servings / **Prep Time:** 15 minutes / **Cooking Time:** 6 minutes)

## Ingredients

- ½ teaspoon fresh ginger, grated
- ¼ teaspoon garlic, minced
- 3 tablespoons soy sauce
- 1 tablespoon red boat fish sauce
- 1 tablespoon fresh lemon juice
- 1 teaspoon Erythritol
- Ground black pepper, as required

- 10½ ounces pork liver, cut into ¼-inch slices
- 2 tablespoons olive oil
- 10 scallions, cut into two-inch lengths

## Instructions

1. In a bowl, mix well ginger, garlic, soy sauce, fish sauce, lemon juice, Erythritol, and black pepper.
2. Add the liver slices and generously coat with the mixture.
3. Cover the bowl and refrigerate to marinate for at least 2 hours.
4. Remove the liver slices from bowl, reserving the marinade.
5. In a large wok, heat the oil and cook liver slices for about 2 minutes, without stirring.
6. Flip and cook for about 1 more minute.
7. Add half of the scallions and reserved marinade and stir fry for about 1-2 minutes.
8. Stir in the remaining scallions and remove from the heat
9. Serve hot.

## Nutrition Values (Per Serving)

- Calories: 273
- Net Carbs: 7.1g
- Carbohydrate: 8.3g
- Fiber: 1.2g
- Protein: 29g
- Fat: 13.9g
- Sugar: 1.3g
- Sodium: 1300mg

---

# Garlicky Pork Shoulder

**(Yields:** 10 servings / **Prep Time:** 15 minutes / **Cooking Time:** 6 hours)

## Ingredients

- 1 head garlic, peeled and crushed
- ¼ cup fresh rosemary, minced
- 2 tablespoons fresh lemon juice
- 2 tablespoons balsamic vinegar
- 1 (4-pound) pork shoulder

## Instructions

1. In a bowl, add all the ingredients except pork shoulder and mix well.
2. In a large roasting pan, place the pork shoulder and generously coat with the marinade.
3. With a large plastic wrap, cover the roasting pan and refrigerate to marinate for at least 1-2 hours.
4. Remove the roasting pan from refrigerator.
5. Remove the plastic wrap from roasting pan and keep in room temperature for 1 hour.

6. Preheat the oven to 275 degrees F.
7. Arrange the roasting pan into oven and roast for about 6 hours.
8. Remove from the oven and place pork shoulder onto a cutting board for about 30 minutes.
9. With a sharp knife, cut the pork shoulder into desired size slices and serve.

## **Nutrition Values (Per Serving)**

- Calories: 502
- Net Carbs: 1.3g
- Carbohydrate: 2g
- Fiber: 0.7g
- Protein: 42.5g
- Fat: 39.1g
- Sugar: 0.1g
- Sodium: 125mg

# **Braised Pork Shoulder**

**(Yields:** 8 servings / **Prep Time:** 15 minutes / **Cooking Time:** 7 hours)

## **Ingredients**

- 3 pounds pork shoulder
- 8 garlic cloves, minced
- ½ cup fresh lemon juice
- 2 tablespoons olive oil
- 1 tablespoon low-sodium soy sauce
- 1/3 cup homemade chicken broth

## **Instructions**

1. In a nonreactive baking dish, arrange the pork shoulder, fat side up.
2. With the tip of knife, score the fat in a crosshatch pattern.
3. In a bowl, mix well garlic, lemon juice, soy sauce and oil.
4. Place the marinade over pork and coat well.
5. Refrigerate for 3-6 hours, flipping occasionally.
6. Preheat the oven to 315 degrees F. Lightly, grease a large roasting pan.
7. With paper towels, wipe marinade off the pork shoulder.
8. Arrange the pork shoulder into prepared roasting pan, fat side up.
9. Roast for about 3 hours.
10. Remove from the oven and add broth over the pork shoulder.
11. Roast for another 3-4 hours, basting with pan juices, after every 1 hour.
12. Remove from oven and place the pork shoulder onto a cutting board for about 30 minutes.
13. With a sharp knife, cut the pork shoulder into desired size slices and serve.

## Nutrition Values (Per Serving)

- Calories: 537
- Net Carbs: 1.4g
- Carbohydrate: 1.5g
- Fiber: 0.1g
- Protein: 40.2g
- Fat: 40.1g
- Sugar: 0.5g
- Sodium: 261mg

**(Tip:** Always choose the shoulder with bone for more flavor.)

---

## Tenderloin with Blueberry Sauce

**(Yields:** 6 servings / **Prep Time:** 15 minutes / **Cooking Time:** 38 minutes)

## Ingredients

### For Pork Tenderloin:

- 3 medium garlic cloves, minced
- 3 teaspoons dried rosemary, crushed
- ½ teaspoon cayenne pepper
- Salt and ground black pepper, as required
- 2 pounds pork tenderloin

### For Blueberry Sauce:

- 1 tablespoon olive oil
- 1 medium yellow onion, chopped
- ½ teaspoon Erythritol
- 1/3 cup organic apple cider vinegar
- 1½ cups fresh blueberries
- ½ teaspoon dried thyme, crushed
- Salt and ground black pepper, as required

## Instructions

1. Preheat the oven to 400 degrees F. Grease a roasting pan.
2. For pork: in a bowl, mix together all the ingredients except pork.
3. Rub the pork evenly with garlic mixture.
4. Place the pork into prepared roasting pan.
5. Roast for about 25 minutes or until desired doneness.
6. Meanwhile, for the sauce; in a pan, heat oil over medium-high heat and sauté the onion for about 4-5 minutes.
7. Stir in the remaining ingredients and cook for about 7-8 minutes or until desired thickness, stirring frequently.
8. Remove the roasting pan from oven and place the pork tenderloin onto a cutting board for about 10-15 minutes.
9. With a sharp knife, cut the pork tenderloin into desired size slices and serve with the topping of blueberry sauce.

## Nutrition Values (Per Serving)

- Calories: 276
- Net Carbs: 7.1g
- Carbohydrate: 8.9g
- Fiber: 1.8g
- Protein: 40.3g
- Fat: 8g
- Sugar: 5.1g
- Sodium: 116mg

===

# Mustard Pork Tenderloin

**(Yields:** 3 servings / **Prep Time:** 15 minutes / **Cooking Time:** 35 minutes)

## Ingredients

- 1 pound pork tenderloin, trimmed
- 3 tablespoons Dijon mustard, divided
- Salt and ground black pepper, as required
- 2 teaspoons olive oil
- ¼ cup organic apple cider vinegar
- 1 teaspoon Erythritol
- 1½ teaspoons fresh sage, chopped

## Instructions

1. Preheat the oven to 425 degrees F.
2. Place the pork tenderloin, 1 tablespoon of Dijon mustard, salt, and black pepper in a bowl and toss to coat well.
3. Heat the oil in a large oven proof wok over medium-high heat and cook the pork tenderloin for about 3-5 minutes or until golden brown from all sides.
4. Immediately, transfer the wok into oven and roast for about 15-20 minutes.
5. Remove the wok from oven and place the pork tenderloin onto a cutting board for about 10-15 minutes.
6. In the same wok, add the vinegar over medium heat and bring to a boil, stirring continuously.
7. Cook for about 1 minute.
8. Stir in the remaining Dijon mustard, and Erythritol and bring to a boil.
9. Immediately, adjust the heat to low and simmer for about 3-5 minutes.
10. With a sharp knife, cut the pork tenderloin into desired size slices and transfer onto serving plates.
11. Top each plate with pan sauce and serve with the garnishing of fresh sage.

## Nutrition Values (Per Serving)

- Calories: 261
- Net Carbs: 0.8g
- Carbohydrate: 1.8g
- Fiber: 1g
- Protein: 40.4g
- Fat: 9.2g
- Sugar: 0.2g
- Sodium: 265mg

# Sweet & Tangy Pork Loin

**(Yields:** 6 servings / **Prep Time:** 15 minutes / **Cooking Time:** 1 hour)

## Ingredients

- 1/3 cup low-sodium soy sauce
- ¼ cup fresh lemon juice
- 2 teaspoons fresh lemon zest, grated
- 1 tablespoon fresh thyme, finely chopped
- 2 tablespoons fresh ginger, grated
- 2 garlic cloves, finely chopped
- 2 tablespoons Erythritol
- Ground black pepper, as required
- ½ teaspoon cayenne pepper
- 2 pounds boneless pork loin

## Instructions

1. For pork marinade: in a large baking dish, add all the ingredients except pork loin and mix until well combined.
2. Add the pork loin and generously coat with the marinade.
3. Refrigerate for about 24 hours.
4. Preheat the oven to 400 degrees F.
5. Remove the pork loin from marinade and arrange into a baking dish.
6. Cover the baking dish and bake for about 1 hour.
7. Remove and place the tenderloins onto a cutting board.
8. With a piece of foil, cover each loin for at least 10 minutes before slicing.
9. With a sharp knife, cut the tenderloins into desired size slices and serve.

## Nutrition Values (Per Serving)

- Calories: 230
- Net Carbs: 2.6g
- Carbohydrate: 3.2g
- Fiber: 0.6g
- Protein: 40.8g
- Fat: 5.6g
- Sugar: 1.2g
- Sodium: 871mg

---

# Creamy Pork Loin

**(Yields:** 2 servings / **Prep Time:** 15 minutes / **Total Cooking Time:** 20 minutes)

## Ingredients

**For Pork Loin:**
- 1 teaspoon dried thyme
- 1 teaspoon paprika
- Salt and ground black pepper, as required
- 4 (4-ounces) pork loins

**For Sauce:**

- ½ cup homemade chicken broth
- ¼ cup heavy cream
- 1 teaspoon organic apple cider vinegar
- 1 tablespoon fresh lemon juice
- 1 tablespoon mustard
- 2 tablespoons fresh parsley, chopped

## Instructions

1. In a small bowl, mix well thyme, paprika, salt, and black pepper.
2. Coat each pork loin evenly with the thyme mixture.
3. Heat a lightly greased large pan over high heat and sear the pork loins for about 2-3 minutes per side.
4. With a slotted spoon, transfer the pork loins onto a plate.
5. In the same pan, add the broth, heavy cream, and vinegar over medium heat and bring to a gentle simmer.
6. Add the lemon juice, and mustard and stir to combine.
7. Stir in the cooked pork loins and simmer, covered partially for about 10 minutes.
8. Garnish with parsley and serve hot.

## Nutrition Values (Per Serving)

- Calories: 647
- Net Carbs: 2.8g
- Carbohydrate: 4.6g
- Fiber: 1.8g
- Protein: 65.4g
- Fat: 39.4g
- Sugar: 0.9g
- Sodium: 342mg

# Sticky Baked Pork Ribs

**(Yields:** 9 servings / **Prep Time:** 15 minutes / **Cooking Time:** 2 hours 34 minutes)

## Ingredients

- ¼ cup Erythritol
- 1 tablespoon garlic powder
- 1 tablespoon paprika
- ½ teaspoon red chili powder
- 4 pounds pork ribs, membrane removed
- Salt and ground black pepper, as required
- 1½ teaspoons liquid smoke
- 1½ cups sugar-free BBQ sauce

## Instructions

1. Preheat the oven to 300 degrees F. Line a large baking sheet with 2 layers of foil, shiny side out.
2. In a bowl, mix well Erythritol, garlic powder, paprika, and chili powder.

3. Season the ribs with salt and black pepper and then, coat with the liquid smoke.
4. Now, rub the ribs evenly with Erythritol mixture.
5. Arrange ribs onto the prepared baking sheet, meaty side down.
6. Arrange 2 layers of foil on top of ribs and then, roll and crimp edges tightly.
7. Bake for about 2-2½ hours or until desired doneness.
8. Remove the baking sheet from oven and place the ribs onto a cutting board.
9. Now, set the oven to broiler.
10. With a sharp knife, cut the ribs into serving sized portions and evenly coat with the barbecue sauce.
11. Arrange the ribs onto a broiler pan, bony side up.
12. Broil for about 1-2 minutes per side.
13. Remove from the oven and serve hot.

## Nutrition Values (Per Serving)

- Calories: 630
- Net Carbs: 2.3g
- Carbohydrate: 2.8g
- Fiber: 0.5g
- Protein: 60.4g
- Fat: 40.3g
- Sugar: 0.4g
- Sodium: 306mg

**(Note:** Make sure to remove the membrane (silver colored skin) from the ribs.)

---

# Spicy Baked Pork Ribs

**(Yields:** 3 servings / **Prep Time:** 15 minutes / **Cooking Time:** 3 hours)

## Ingredients

- 1 teaspoon garlic powder
- 1 teaspoon onion powder
- 1 teaspoon red chili powder
- ½ teaspoon cayenne pepper
- ½ teaspoon smoked paprika
- Salt and ground black pepper, as required
- 1 pound baby back ribs rack, membrane removed

## Instructions

1. Preheat the oven to 275 degrees F. Line a baking sheet with parchment paper.
2. In a small bowl, mix well all the spices, salt and black pepper.
3. Rub the ribs evenly with spice mixture.
4. Arrange the ribs onto prepared baking sheet.
5. Bake for about 3 hours.
6. Remove from the oven and place ribs onto a cutting board for about 5 minutes.
7. Cut the rack into individual rib segments and serve.

### Nutrition Values (Per Serving)

- Calories: 350
- Net Carbs: 1.7g
- Carbohydrate: 2.6g
- Fiber: 0.9g
- Protein: 40.4g
- Fat: 18.8g
- Sugar: 0.7g
- Sodium: 892mg

**(Note:** You can serve this with your favorite sugar-free barbecue sauce.)

---

## Cheesy Pork Cutlets

**(Yields:** 6 servings / **Prep Time:** 15 minutes / **Total Cooking Time:** 20 minutes)

### Ingredients

- ½ cup Italian dressing
- ½ cup Parmesan cheese, grated
- 1 tablespoon pork seasoning
- 6 (6-ounces) pork cutlets
- 2 tablespoons butter, divided

### Instructions

1. Add the Italian dressing in a shallow dish.
2. Add the cheese and seasoning in another dish and mix well.
3. Dip each pork cutlet with Italian dressing and then, coat with the parmesan mixture.
4. Melt 1 tablespoon of butter in a large wok over medium heat and cook 3 cutlets for about 5 minutes per side.
5. Repeat with the remaining butter and cutlets.
6. Serve hot.

### Nutrition Values (Per Serving)

- Calories: 326
- Net Carbs: 2g
- Carbohydrate: 2g
- Fiber: 0g
- Protein: 40.4g
- Fat: 17g
- Sugar: 1.6g
- Sodium: 189mg

---

## Sweet & Sour Pork Chops

**(Yields:** 6 servings / **Prep Time:** 15 minutes / **Cooking Time:** 50 minutes)

### Ingredients

- 6 (8-ounces) (¾-inch thick) pork shoulder chops, trimmed
- Salt and ground black pepper, as required

- 2 tablespoons olive oil
- 1¼ cups water
- ¾ cup organic apple cider vinegar
- 6 garlic cloves, mashed
- 2 tablespoons Erythritol
- 2 tablespoons fresh parsley, minced

## Instructions

1. Preheat the oven to 400 degrees F.
2. Season each chop evenly with salt and black pepper.
3. In a large Dutch oven, heat the oil over high heat and sear the chops in 2 batches for about 5 minutes, flipping once halfway through.
4. Remove the pan from heat and arrange the chops in a single layer.
5. In a bowl, add the remaining ingredients except parsley and mix well.
6. Add the vinegar mixture evenly over chops.
7. Cover the pan and transfer into oven.
8. Bake for about 40 minutes.
9. Garnish with parsley and serve hot.

## Nutrition Values (Per Serving)

- Calories: 777
- Net Carbs: 1.3g
- Carbohydrate: 1.4g
- Fiber: 0.1g
- Protein: 51.2g
- Fat: 61.1g
- Sugar: 0.2g
- Sodium: 189mg

---

# Parmesan Pork Chops

(**Yields:** 4 servings / **Prep Time:** 15 minutes / **Cooking Time:** 25 minutes)

## Ingredients

- ¾ cup parmesan cheese, shredded
- 4 tablespoons butter, melted
- 6 garlic cloves, minced
- ½ tablespoon fresh thyme, minced
- ½ tablespoon fresh parsley, minced
- Salt and ground black pepper, as required
- 8 (3-ounces) center-cut thin boneless pork chops

## Instructions

1. Preheat the oven to 400 degrees F. Line a baking dish with a greased parchment paper.
2. In a bowl, mix together the cheese, butter, garlic, herbs, salt, and black pepper.
3. Arrange the pork chops into prepared baking dish in a single layer.
4. Coat the chops evenly with parmesan mixture.

5. Bake for about 20-25 minutes.
6. Remove the baking dish from oven and set the oven to broiler.
7. Broil the chops for about 3 minutes.
8. Remove from the oven and serve hot.

## Nutrition Values (Per Serving)

- Calories: 415
- Net Carbs: 2.1g
- Carbohydrate: 2.3g
- Fiber: 0.2g
- Protein: 50.7g
- Fat: 21.6g
- Sugar: 0.1g
- Sodium: 473mg

---

# Basil Pork Chops

**(Yields:** 4 servings / **Prep Time:** 15 minutes / **Cooking Time:** 12 minutes)

## Ingredients

- 1 cup fresh basil leaves, minced
- 2 garlic cloves, minced
- 2 tablespoons olive oil
- 2 tablespoons fresh lemon juice
- Salt and ground black pepper, as required
- 4 (6-8-ounces) bone-in pork loin chops

## Instructions

1. In a baking dish, mix well basil, garlic, oil, lemon juice, salt, and black pepper.
2. Add the chops and generously coat with the mixture.
3. Cover and refrigerate for about 30-45 minutes.
4. Preheat a gas grill to medium-high heat. Lightly, grease the grill grate.
5. Place chops onto a grill and cook for about 6 minutes per side or until desired doneness.
6. Serve hot.

## Nutrition Values (Per Serving)

- Calories: 426
- Net Carbs: 2.5g
- Carbohydrate: 2.7g
- Fiber: 0.2g
- Protein: 43.9g
- Fat: 25.1g
- Sugar: 1.7g
- Sodium: 378mg

# Spiced Pork Chops

**(Yields:** 4 servings / **Prep Time:** 15 minutes / **Cooking Time:** 12 minutes)

## Ingredients

- 2 tablespoons olive oil
- 1 tablespoon Worcestershire sauce
- 1 teaspoon fresh lemon juice
- 1 teaspoon paprika
- ½ teaspoon onion powder
- ½ teaspoon ground cumin
- ½ teaspoon garlic paste
- Salt and ground black pepper, as required
- 4 (6-ounces) boneless pork chops

## Instructions

1. In a large baking dish, mix well all the ingredients except chops.
2. Add the chops and generously coat with the mixture.
3. Cover and set aside at room temperature for about 10-15 minutes.
4. Heat a greased grill pan over medium-high heat and cook the chops for about 4-6 minutes per side.
5. Serve hot.

## Nutrition Values (Per Serving)

- Calories: 311
- Net Carbs: 1.3g
- Carbohydrate: 1.6g
- Fiber: 0.3g
- Protein: 44.7g
- Fat: 13.1g
- Sugar: 1g
- Sodium: 178mg

---

# Buttered Pork Chops

**(Yields:** 4 servings / **Prep Time:** 15 minutes / **Total Cooking Time:** 12 minutes)

## Ingredients

- 4 (6-ounces) boneless pork chops
- Salt and ground black pepper, as required
- 3 tablespoons unsalted butter
- 1 tablespoon fresh parsley
- 1 teaspoon garlic, minced
- 2 teaspoons fresh lemon juice

## Instructions

1. Season each chop evenly with salt and black pepper.
2. Melt the butter in a wok over medium-high heat and sauté the parsley and garlic for about 20-30 seconds.
3. Stir in the chops and cook for about 5 minutes per side or until cooked through, stirring frequently.
4. Add in the lemon juice and remove from heat.
5. Serve hot.

### Nutrition Values (Per Serving)
- Calories: 322
- Net Carbs: 0.3g
- Carbohydrate: 0.4g
- Fiber: 0.1g
- Protein: 44.7g
- Fat: 14.6g
- Sugar: 0.1g
- Sodium: 198mg

=====================================================

## Stuffed Pork Chops

**(Yields:** 4 servings / **Prep Time:** 20 minutes / **Cooking Time:** 1 hour 5 minutes)

### Ingredients
- 3 bacon slices, chopped
- 4 (6-ounces) boneless pork chops
- 3 ounces feta cheese, crumbled
- 3 ounces blue cheese, crumbled
- 2 ounces cream cheese
- 4 medium scallions, chopped
- Salt and ground black pepper, as required

### Instructions
1. Preheat the oven to 350 degrees F. Grease a baking dish.
2. Heat a wok over medium-high heat and cook the bacon for about 6-7 minutes.
3. With a slotted spoon, transfer the bacon into a bowl, leaving the grease in wok.
4. In the bowl of bacon, mix well feta cheese, blue cheese, cream cheese and scallion.
5. With a sharp knife, cut a slit into each pork chop horizontally, making a pocket for the filling.
6. Stuff each pork chop with the cheese mixture and then, secure with toothpicks.
7. Rub the outside of pork chops with salt and black pepper.
8. Heat the same wok with bacon grease over high heat and sear the pork chops for about 1½ minutes per side.
9. Remove from heat and arrange the chops into prepared baking dish in a single layer.
10. Bake for about 55 minutes or until desired doneness.
11. Remove from oven and set the pork chops aside for about 3 minutes before serving.

### Nutrition Values (Per Serving)
- Calories: 546
- Net Carbs: 2.8g
- Carbohydrate: 3.2g
- Fiber: 0.4g
- Protein: 61.5g
- Fat: 30.7g
- Sugar: 1.4g
- Sodium: 1200mg

# Stuffed Pork Tenderloin

**(Yields:** 3 servings / **Prep Time:** 20 minutes / **Cooking Time:** 1 hour 20 minutes)

## Ingredients

- 1 pound pork tenderloin
- 1 tablespoon unsalted butter
- 2 teaspoons garlic, minced
- 2 ounces fresh spinach
- 4 ounces cream cheese, softened
- 1 teaspoon liquid smoke
- Salt and ground black pepper, as required

## Instructions

1. Preheat the oven to 350 degrees F. Line casserole dish with a piece of foil.
2. Arrange the pork tenderloin between 2 plastic wraps and with a meat tenderizer, pound until flat.
3. Carefully, cut the edges of tenderloin to shape into a rectangle.
4. Melt the butter in a large wok over medium heat and sauté the garlic for about 1 minute.
5. Add the spinach, cream cheese, liquid smoke, salt, and black pepper and cook for about 3-4 minutes.
6. Remove the wok from heat and let it cool slightly.
7. Place the spinach mixture onto pork tenderloin about ½-inch from the edges.
8. Carefully, roll tenderloin into a log and secure with toothpicks.
9. Arrange tenderloin into the prepared casserole dish, seam-side down.
10. Bake for about 1¼ hours.
11. Remove the casserole dish from oven and let it cool slightly before cutting.
12. Cut the tenderloin into desired size slices and serve.

## Nutrition Values (Per Serving)

- Calories: 389
- Net Carbs: 1.8g
- Carbohydrate: 2.3g
- Fiber: 0.5g
- Protein: 43.1g
- Fat: 22.4g
- Sugar: 0.2g
- Sodium: 291mg

# Bacon Wrapped Pork Tenderloin

**(Yields:** 6 servings / **Prep Time:** 20 minutes / **Cooking Time:** 35 minutes)

## Ingredients

- 8 bacon slices
- 2 pounds pork tenderloin
- 1 teaspoon dried oregano, crushed
- 1 teaspoon dried basil, crushed
- 1 tablespoon garlic powder
- 1 teaspoon seasoned salt
- 3 tablespoons butter

## Instructions

1. Preheat the oven to 400 degrees F.
2. Heat a large ovenproof wok over medium-high heat and cook the bacon for about 6-7 minutes.
3. Transfer the bacon onto a paper towel-lined plate to drain.
4. Wrap the pork tenderloin with bacon slices and secure with toothpicks.
5. With a sharp knife, slice the tenderloins between each bacon slice to make a medallion.
6. In a bowl, mix well dried herbs, garlic powder and seasoned salt.
7. Now, coat the wrapped pork evenly with herb mixture.
8. With a paper towel, wipe out the same wok.
9. In the wok, melt the butter over medium-high heat and cook the pork for about 4 minutes per side.
10. Now, transfer the wok into oven.
11. Roast for about 17-20 minutes.
12. Remove the wok from oven and let it cool slightly before cutting.
13. Cut the tenderloin into desired size slices and serve.

## Nutrition Values (Per Serving)

- Calories: 471
- Net Carbs: 0.8g
- Carbohydrate: 1g
- Fiber: 0.2g
- Protein: 53.5g
- Fat: 26.6g
- Sugar: 0.1g
- Sodium: 1100mg

---

# Ground Pork with Greens

**(Yields:** 4 servings / **Prep Time:** 15 minutes / **Cooking Time:** 20 minutes)

## Ingredients

- 1 tablespoon olive oil
- ½ of yellow onion, chopped
- 2 garlic cloves, finely chopped
- 1 jalapeño pepper, finely chopped
- 1-pound lean ground pork
- 1 teaspoon ground coriander
- 1 teaspoon ground cumin
- ½ teaspoon ground turmeric
- Salt and ground black pepper, as required
- ¾ pound collard greens leaves, stemmed and chopped
- 8 fresh cherry tomatoes, quartered
- 1 teaspoon fresh lemon juice

## Instructions

1. Heat the oil in a large wok over medium heat and sauté the onion for about 4-5 minutes.
2. Add the garlic, and jalapeño pepper and sauté for about 1 minute.

3. Add the pork, spices, salt, and black pepper and cook for about 6-8 minutes.
4. Stir in the collard greens, and tomatoes and cook for about 4-5 minutes, stirring frequently.
5. Add lemon juice and remove from the heat.
6. Serve hot.

## **Nutrition Values (Per Serving)**

- Calories: 306
- Net Carbs: 5.3g
- Carbohydrate: 9.3g
- Fiber: 4g
- Protein: 22.1g
- Fat: 21.4g
- Sugar: 2.3g
- Sodium: 58mg

**(Note:** You can replace cherry tomatoes with grape tomatoes.)

---

# **Pork & Spinach Meatloaf**

**(Yields:** 8 servings / **Prep Time:** 1 minutes / **Cooking Time:** 1¼ hours)

## **Ingredients**

- 2 pounds ground pork
- ½ cup yellow onion, chopped
- ½ cup green bell pepper, seeded and chopped
- 2 garlic cloves, minced
- 1 cup cheddar cheese, grated
- ¼ cup sugar-free ketchup
- ¼ cup sugar-free HP steak sauce
- 2 organic eggs, beaten
- 1 teaspoon dried thyme, crushed
- Salt and ground black pepper, as required
- 3 cups fresh spinach, chopped
- 2 cups mozzarella cheese, grated freshly

## **Instructions**

1. Preheat the oven to 350 degrees F. Lightly, grease a baking dish.
2. In a large bowl, add all the ingredients except spinach, and mozzarella cheese and mix until well combined.
3. Place a large wax paper onto a smooth surface.
4. Place the meat mixture over wax paper.
5. Add the spinach over meat mixture, pressing slightly.
6. Top with the mozzarella cheese.
7. Roll the wax paper around meat mixture to form a meatloaf.
8. Carefully, remove the wax paper and place meatloaf onto the prepared baking dish.
9. Bake for about 1-1¼ hours.
10. Remove from the oven and set aside for about 10 minutes before serving.
11. With a sharp knife, cut into desired size slices and serve.

## Nutrition Values (Per Serving)

- Calories: 300
- Net Carbs: 5.9g
- Carbohydrate: 6.6g
- Fiber: 0.7g
- Protein: 34g
- Fat: 14.1g
- Sugar: 4g
- Sodium: 323mg

---

# Pork Pinwheel

(**Yields:** 10 servings / **Prep Time:** 15 minutes / **Cooking Time:** 40 minutes)

## Ingredients

**For Meatloaf:**

- 2 pounds ground pork
- 1 cup cheddar cheese, shredded
- 1 tablespoon dried onion, minced
- 1 teaspoon dried garlic, minced
- 1 teaspoon red chili powder
- 1 teaspoon garlic powder
- 1 teaspoon ground mustard
- Salt, as required
- 1 organic egg, beaten
- 2 ounces sugar-free BBQ sauce

**For Topping:**

- 2 ounces sugar-free BBQ sauce
- 5 cooked bacon slices, chopped
- ½ cup cheddar cheese, shredded

## Instructions

1. Preheat the oven to 400 degrees F. Grease a 9x13-inch casserole dish.
2. For meatloaf: add all the ingredients in a bowl and mix until well combined.
3. Place the mixture evenly into prepared casserole dish and press to smooth the surface.
4. Coat the top of meatloaf evenly with BBQ sauce and sprinkle with bacon, followed by cheese.
5. Bake for approximately 40 minutes.
6. Remove the meatloaf from oven and keep onto a wire rack to cool slightly.
7. Cut the meatloaf into desired size slices and serve warm.

## Nutrition Values (Per Serving)

- Calories: 244
- Net Carbs: 0.9g
- Carbohydrate: 1.6g
- Fiber: 0.7g
- Protein: 31.3g
- Fat: 11.7g
- Sugar: 0.2g
- Sodium: 515mg

# Pork Casserole

**(Yields:** 8 servings / **Prep Time:** 20 minutes / **Cooking Time:** 55 minutes)

## Ingredients

- 1 pound pork sausage
- ½ pound fresh mushrooms, sliced
- 1 celery stalk, finely chopped
- 1 tablespoon onion, chopped
- 8 ounces cream cheese, softened
- 4 cups cooked pork, chopped
- 8 ounces cheddar cheese, shredded
- 16 ounces frozen cauliflower, boiled, drained and roughly chopped
- Salt and ground black pepper, as required
- 1/8 teaspoon paprika

## Instructions

1. Preheat the oven to 350 degrees F. Grease a 13x9-inch casserole dish.
2. Heat a large nonstick wok over medium heat and cook the sausage, mushroom, celery, and onion for about 8-10 minutes, stirring frequently.
3. Add the cream cheese and stir to combine well.
4. Stir in the pork, cheddar cheese, cauliflower, salt, and black pepper and remove from the heat.
5. Transfer the mixture evenly into prepared casserole dish and sprinkle with paprika.
6. Cover the baking dish and bake for about 30 minutes.
7. Uncover and bake for about 10-15 more minutes or until top becomes golden brown.
8. Remove from the oven and set aside for about 5 minutes before serving.
9. Cut into desired size pieces and serve.

## Nutrition Values (Per Serving)

- Calories: 534
- Net Carbs: 3.5g
- Carbohydrate: 5.3g
- Fiber: 1.8g
- Protein: 41.9g
- Fat: 38.1g
- Sugar: 2.1g
- Sodium: 767mg

# CHAPTER 5 | POULTRY

## Roasted Whole Chicken

**(Yields:** 4 servings / **Prep Time:** 20 minutes / **Cooking Time:** 1 hour 32 minutes)

### Ingredients

- 10 tablespoons unsalted butter
- 3 garlic cloves, minced
- 1 (3-pounds) grass-fed whole chicken, neck and giblets removed
- Salt and ground black pepper, as required

### Instructions

1. Preheat the oven to 400 degrees F. Arrange an oven rack into the lower portion of oven.
2. Grease a large baking dish.
3. Place the butter and garlic in a small pan over medium heat and cook for about 1-2 minutes.
4. Remove the pan from heat and let it cool for about 2 minutes.
5. Season the inside and outside of chicken evenly with salt and black pepper.
6. Arrange the chicken into prepared baking dish, breast side up.
7. Pour the garlic butter over and inside of the chicken.
8. Bake for about 1-1½ hours, basting with the pan juices after every 20 minutes.
9. Remove from oven and place the chicken onto a cutting board for about 5-10 minutes before carving.
10. Cut into desired size pieces and serve.

### Nutrition Values (Per Serving)

- Calories: 772
- Net Carbs: 0.7g
- Carbohydrate: 0.8g
- Fiber: 0.1g
- Protein: 99g
- Fat: 39.1g
- Sugar: 0g
- Sodium: 458mg

---

## Grilled Whole Chicken

**(Yields:** 6 servings / **Prep Time:** 20 minutes / **Cooking Time:** 20 minutes)

### Ingredients

- ¼ cup olive oil
- 2 tablespoons fresh lemon juice
- 2 teaspoons fresh lemon zest, grated finely

- 1 teaspoon dried oregano, crushed
- 2 teaspoons paprika
- 1 teaspoon onion powder
- 1 teaspoon garlic powder
- Salt and ground black pepper, as required
- 1 (4-pounds) grass-fed whole chicken, neck and giblets removed

## Instructions

1. Preheat the grill to medium heat. Grease the grill grate.
2. Add the oil, lemon juice, lemon zest, oregano, spices, salt, and black pepper in a bowl and mix until well combined.
3. Place the chicken on a cutting board, breast side down.
4. With a sharp knife, cut along both sides of backbone and then remove the backbone.
5. Flip the breast side up and open it like a book.
6. With the palm of your hands, firmly press breast to flatten.
7. Generously, coat the whole chicken with oil mixture.
8. Arrange chicken onto the grill and cook for about 16-20 minutes, flipping once halfway through.
9. Remove from grill and place the chicken onto a cutting board for about 5-10 minutes before carving.
10. Cut into desired size pieces and serve.

## Nutrition Values (Per Serving)

- Calories: 654
- Net Carbs: 1g
- Carbohydrate: 1.5g
- Fiber: 0.5g
- Protein: 87.8g
- Fat: 31g
- Sugar: 0.5g
- Sodium: 289mg

---

# Roasted Spatchcock Chicken

**(Yields:** 6 servings / **Prep Time:** 20 minutes / **Cooking Time:** 50 minutes)

## Ingredients

- 1 (4-pounds) grass-fed whole chicken, neck and giblets removed
- 1 (1-inch) piece fresh ginger, sliced
- 4 garlic cloves, chopped
- 1 small bunch fresh thyme
- Pinch of cayenne pepper
- Salt and ground black pepper, as required
- ¼ cup fresh lemon juice
- 3 tablespoons olive oil

## Instructions

1. Arrange the chicken onto a large cutting board, breast side down.

2. With a kitchen shear, start from thigh and cut along 1 side of the backbone and turn chicken around.
3. Now, cut along the other side and discard the backbone.
4. Change the side and open it like a book and then, flatten the backbone firmly.
5. Place the remaining ingredients in a food processor and pulse until smooth.
6. In a large baking dish, add the marinade mixture.
7. Add the chicken and generously coat with marinade.
8. With a plastic wrap, cover the baking dish and refrigerate to marinate overnight.
9. Preheat the oven to 450 degrees F. Arrange a lightly greased rack into a roasting pan.
10. Remove the chicken from refrigerator and place onto the rack over roasting pan, skin side down.
11. Roast for about 50 minutes, flipping once halfway through.
12. Remove from oven and place the chicken onto a platter for about 10-15 minutes before carving.
13. With a sharp knife, cut the chicken into desired size pieces and serve.

## Nutrition Values (Per Serving)

- Calories: 523
- Net Carbs: 1g
- Carbohydrate: 1.2g
- Fiber: 0.2g
- Protein: 87.7g
- Fat: 29.5g
- Sugar: 0.2g
- Sodium: 290mg

**(Tip:** Feel free to add more seasonings and spices if you like spicy chicken.)

---

# Stuffed Cornish Hens

**(Yields:** 8 servings / **Prep Time:** 20 minutes / **Cooking Time:** 1 hour)

## Ingredients

- 1 tablespoon dried basil, crushed
- 2 tablespoons lemon pepper
- 1 tablespoon poultry seasoning
- Salt, to taste
- 4 (1½-pounds) grass-fed Cornish game hens, rinsed and dried completely
- 2 tablespoons olive oil
- 1 yellow onion, chopped
- 1 celery stalk, chopped
- 1 green bell pepper, seeded and chopped

## Instructions

1. Preheat the oven to 375 degrees F. Arrange lightly greased racks in 2 large roasting pans.
2. In a bowl, mix well basil, lemon pepper, poultry seasoning, and salt.
3. Coat each hen with oil and then, rub evenly with the seasoning mixture.
4. In a next bowl, mix together the onion, celery and bell pepper.
5. Stuff the cavity of each hen loosely with veggie mixture.
6. Arrange the hens into prepared roasting pans, keeping plenty of space between them.
7. Roast for about 1 hour or until the juices run clear.
8. Remove the hens from oven and place onto a cutting board.
9. With a foil piece, cover each hen loosely for about 10 minutes before carving.
10. Cut into desired size pieces and serve.

## Nutrition Values (Per Serving)

- Calories: 714
- Net Carbs: 2.8g
- Carbohydrate: 3.8g
- Fiber: 1g
- Protein: 58.2g
- Fat: 52.2g
- Sugar: 1.4g
- Sodium: 235mg

---

# Parmesan Chicken Drumsticks

**(Yields:** 6 servings / **Prep Time:** 15 minutes / **Cooking Time:** 45 minutes)

## Ingredients

- ½ cup Parmesan cheese, grated freshly
- 1 teaspoon garlic, minced
- 1 teaspoon dried onion, minced
- 1 teaspoon dried basil
- 1 teaspoon dried oregano
- 1 teaspoon dried parsley
- Salt and ground black pepper, as required
- 6 (6-ounces) grass-fed chicken drumsticks
- Olive oil cooking spray

## Instructions

1. Preheat the oven to 425 degrees F. Grease a large baking sheet.
2. Add the parmesan cheese, garlic, onion, herbs, salt, and black pepper in a bowl and mix well.
3. With wet fingers, wet each chicken drumsticks slightly.
4. With your hands, pat the cheese mixture evenly onto each chicken drumstick and then, spray with the cooking spray.
5. Arrange the chicken drumstick onto prepared baking sheet in a single layer.

6. Bake for about 45 minutes, flipping twice.
7. Remove from the oven and serve hot.

## Nutrition Values (Per Serving)

- Calories: 313
- Net Carbs: 0.3g
- Carbohydrate: 0.4g
- Fiber: 0.1g
- Protein: 49.5g
- Fat: 11.3g
- Sugar: 0g
- Sodium: 221mg

---

# Glazed Chicken Thighs

**(Yields:** 4 servings / **Prep Time:** 15 minutes / **Total Cooking Time:** 20 minutes)

## Ingredients

- 1 small yellow onion, minced
- 2 garlic cloves, minced
- 2 tablespoons fresh cilantro, minced
- 1/3 cup sugar-free ketchup
- 1/3 cup low-sodium soy sauce
- 2½ tablespoons organic apple cider vinegar
- 1 tablespoon olive oil
- 2 packets stevia
- 1 teaspoon red pepper flakes, crushed
- Ground black pepper, as required
- 4 (6-ounces) grass-fed skinless, boneless chicken thighs

## Instructions

1. Add all the ingredients except chicken thighs into a glass baking dish and mix well.
2. Add the chicken thighs and generously, coat with the mixture.
3. Refrigerate overnight.
4. Preheat the broiler of oven. Line a large baking sheet with a greased piece of foil.
5. Remove the chicken thighs from bowl, reserving the remaining marinade.
6. Arrange the chicken thighs onto prepared baking sheet in a single layer and broil for about 5 minutes per side.
7. Meanwhile, transfer the reserved marinade into a small pan over medium heat and cook for about 8-10 minutes.
8. Serve the chicken thighs alongside the sauce.

## Nutrition Values (Per Serving)

- Calories: 304
- Net Carbs: 6.8g
- Carbohydrate: 7.3g
- Fiber: 0.5g
- Protein: 39.6g
- Fat: 13g
- Sugar: 2.1g
- Sodium: 1310mg

# Tangy Chicken Breasts

**(Yields:** 4 servings / **Prep Time:** 15 minutes / **Cooking Time:** 14 minutes)

## Ingredients

- ¼ cup balsamic vinegar
- 2 tablespoons butter, melted
- 1½ teaspoons fresh lemon juice
- ½ teaspoon lemon-pepper seasoning
- 4 (6-ounces) grass-fed boneless, skinless chicken breast halves, pounded slightly

## Instructions

1. Place the vinegar, butter, lemon juice and seasoning into a glass baking dish and mix well.
2. Add the chicken breasts and generously, coat with the mixture.
3. Refrigerate to marinate for about 25-30 minutes.
4. Preheat the grill to medium heat. Grease the grill grate.
5. Remove the chicken from bowl and discard the remaining marinade.
6. Place the chicken breasts onto grill and cover with the lid.
7. Cook for about 5-7 minutes per side or until desired doneness.
8. Serve hot.

## Nutrition Values (Per Serving)

- Calories: 378
- Net Carbs: 0.3g
- Carbohydrate: 0.4g
- Fiber: 0.1g
- Protein: 49.3g
- Fat: 18.4g
- Sugar: 0.1g
- Sodium: 188mg

# Spicy Chicken Leg Quarters

**(Yields:** 3 servings / **Prep Time:** 15 minutes / **Cooking Time:** 53 minutes)

## Ingredients

- 3 (10-11 ounces) grass-fed bone-in, skin-on chicken leg quarters
- ½ cup mayonnaise
- 1 teaspoon paprika
- ½ teaspoon garlic powder
- Salt and ground white pepper, as required

## Instructions

1. Preheat the oven to 350 degrees. Generously, grease a baking dish.
2. Add the mayonnaise in a shallow bowl.

3. Place the paprika, garlic powder, salt and white pepper in a small bowl and mix well.
4. Coat each chicken quarter with mayonnaise and then, sprinkle evenly with the spice mixture.
5. Arrange the chicken quarters onto prepared baking sheet in a single layer.
6. Bake for about 45 minutes.
7. Now, increase the temperature of oven to 400 degrees F and bake for about 5-8 more minutes.
8. Remove from oven and place the chicken quarters onto a platter.
9. With a piece of foil, cover each chicken quarter loosely for about 5-10 minutes before serving.
10. Serve.

## Nutrition Values (Per Serving)

- Calories: 725
- Net Carbs: 0.4g
- Carbohydrate: 0.7g
- Fiber: 0.3g
- Protein: 48.3g
- Fat: 59.7g
- Sugar: 0.2g
- Sodium: 746mg

---

## Chicken Chili

**(Yields:** 4 servings / **Prep Time:** 15 minutes / **Cooking Time:** 1 hour**)**

## Ingredients

- 3 tablespoons unsalted butter
- 1 pound grass-fed chicken breasts
- ¼ cup yellow onion, chopped
- 1 green bell pepper, seeded and chopped
- 2 garlic cloves, minced
- 3 ounces canned chopped green chiles, drained
- 1 jalapeño pepper, chopped
- 1 teaspoon dried oregano
- 1 teaspoon ground cumin
- 1 teaspoon red chili powder
- ¼ teaspoon cayenne pepper
- Salt and ground white pepper, as required
- 1½ cups homemade chicken broth
- 4 ounces cream cheese, softened
- ¼ cup heavy whipping cream
- ¼ cup Pepper Jack cheese, shredded

## Instructions

1. Melt the butter into a large pan over medium heat and cook the chicken breasts for about 3-4 minutes per side.
2. With a slotted spoon, transfer the chicken breasts onto a plate.
3. In the same pan, add the onion, and bell pepper and sauté for about 5-6 minutes.

4. Add the garlic, green chiles, jalapeño pepper, herbs, spices, salt, and black pepper and sauté for about 1 minute.
5. Stir in the cooked chicken breasts, and broth and bring to a boil.
6. Adjust the heat to medium-low and simmer, covered for about 30 minutes.
7. With a slotted spoon, transfer the chicken breasts into a bowl and with 2 forks, shred the meat.
8. Return the shredded meat into pan and stir to combine.
9. Stir in the cream cheese, and cream and cook for about 10-15 more minutes.
10. Top with the Pepper Jack cheese and serve hot.

## **Nutrition Values (Per Serving)**
- Calories: 484
- Net Carbs: 6.3g
- Carbohydrate: 7.5g
- Fiber: 1.2g
- Protein: 39.3g
- Fat: 32.6g
- Sugar: 3.1g
- Sodium: 735mg

## **Butter Chicken**

(**Yields:** 5 servings / **Prep Time:** 15 minutes / **Cooking Time:** 25 minutes)

## **Ingredients**
- 2 tablespoons unsalted butter
- 1 medium yellow onion, chopped
- 2 garlic cloves, minced
- 1 teaspoon fresh ginger, minced
- 1½ pounds grass-fed chicken breasts, cut into ¾-inch chunks
- 1 (6-ounces) can sugar-free tomato paste
- 1 tablespoon garam masala
- 1 teaspoon red chili powder
- 1 teaspoon ground cumin
- Salt and ground black pepper, as required
- 1 cup heavy cream
- 2 tablespoons fresh cilantro, chopped

## **Instructions**
1. Melt the butter in a large skillet over medium-high heat and sauté the onions for about 5-6 minutes.
2. Add the garlic, and ginger and sauté for about 1 minute.
3. Stir in the chicken, tomato paste, spices, salt, and black pepper and cook for about 6-8 minutes or until desired doneness of the chicken.
4. Stir in the heavy cream and cook for about 8-10 more minutes, stirring occasionally.
5. Garnish with fresh cilantro and serve hot.

### Nutrition Values (Per Serving)

- Calories: 425
- Net Carbs: 7.8g
- Carbohydrate: 10.1g
- Fiber: 2.3g
- Protein: 41.9g
- Fat: 24g
- Sugar: 4g
- Sodium: 233mg

(**Tip:** You can replace the tomato paste with tomato puree if you desired.)

---

# Spicy Chicken Curry

(**Yields:** 6 servings / **Prep Time:** 15 minutes / **Cooking Time:** 30 minutes)

## Ingredients

- 2 tablespoons olive oil
- 1 yellow onion, chopped
- 1 tablespoon garlic, minced
- ½ tablespoon fresh ginger, grated finely
- 1 tablespoon curry powder
- 1 teaspoon ground coriander
- 1 teaspoon ground cumin
- ½ teaspoon paprika
- ½ teaspoon cayenne pepper
- 6 (4-ounces) grass-fed skinless, boneless chicken thighs, cut into 1-inch pieces
- 3 Roma tomatoes, finely chopped
- 8 ounces unsweetened coconut milk
- 8 ounces homemade chicken broth
- Salt and ground black pepper, as required
- ¼ cup fresh cilantro, chopped

## Instructions

1. Heat the oil in a large nonstick pan over medium heat and sauté the onion for about 8-9 minutes, stirring frequently.
2. Add the garlic, ginger and spices and sauté for about 1 minute.
3. Stir in the chicken pieces and cook for about 4-5 minutes.
4. Add the tomatoes, coconut milk, broth, salt, and black pepper and bring to a gentle simmer.
5. Adjust the heat to low and simmer, covered for about 10-15 minutes or until desired doneness.
6. Stir in cilantro and remove from the heat.
7. Serve hot.

## Nutrition Values (Per Serving)

- Calories: 300
- Net Carbs: 5.3g
- Carbohydrate: 7.6g
- Fiber: 2.3g
- Protein: 28g
- Fat: 18.3g
- Sugar: 3.9g
- Sodium: 199mg

# Chicken in Cheesy Buffalo Sauce

**(Yields:** 4 servings / **Prep Time:** 15 minutes / **Total Cooking Time:** 18 minutes)

## Ingredients

- 4 (4-ounces) boneless, skinless chicken breasts
- 1 teaspoon garlic powder
- Salt and ground black pepper, as required
- 3 tablespoons unsalted butter, divided
- 2 garlic cloves, minced
- 1 cup sugar-free buffalo sauce
- Pinch of cayenne pepper
- 8 muenster cheese slices
- 2 tablespoons fresh chives, chopped

## Instructions

1. Season each chicken breast evenly with garlic powder, salt and black pepper.
2. Melt 1 tablespoon of butter in a large skillet over medium heat and cook the chicken breasts for about 5-7 minutes per side.
3. With a slotted spoon, transfer the chicken breasts onto a plate.
4. Now, melt the remaining butter in the same skillet over medium heat and sauté the garlic for about 1 minute.
5. Add the buffalo sauce and cayenne pepper and stir to combine.
6. Stir in the cooked chicken breasts and top each with 2 cheese slices.
7. Simmer, covered for about 3 minutes.
8. Garnish with fresh chives and serve hot.

## Nutrition Values (Per Serving)

- Calories: 612
- Net Carbs: 1.8g
- Carbohydrate: 2g
- Fiber: 0.2g
- Protein: 62.7g
- Fat: 38.1g
- Sugar: 0.9g
- Sodium: 694mg

---

# Chicken in Capers Sauce

**(Yield:** 2 servings / **Prep Time:** 15 minutes / **Cooking Time:** 25 minutes)

## Ingredients

- 2 (5½ oz.) grass-fed boneless, skinless chicken thighs, cut in half horizontally
- Salt and ground black pepper, as required
- 1/3 cup almond flour

- 2 tablespoons Parmesan cheese, shredded
- ½ teaspoon garlic powder
- 2 tablespoons butter, divided
- 1 tablespoon garlic, minced
- 3 tablespoons capers
- ¼ teaspoon red pepper flakes, crushed
- 3-4 tablespoons fresh lemon juice
- 1 cup homemade chicken broth
- 1/3 cup heavy cream
- 2 tablespoons fresh parsley, chopped

## Instructions

1. Coat the chicken thighs evenly with salt and black pepper.
2. In a shallow dish, mix well flour, parmesan cheese and garlic powder.
3. Coat the chicken thighs with flour mixture and then shake off any excess.
4. Melt 1 tablespoon of butter in a large skillet over medium-high heat and cook the chicken thighs for about 4-5 minutes per side.
5. With a slotted spoon, place the chicken thighs onto a platter and with a piece of foil, cover them to keep warm.
6. In a bowl, add the capers, garlic, red pepper flakes, lemon juice, and broth and beat until well combined.
7. Melt the remaining butter in the same skillet over medium heat and with a spoon, scrape the brown bits from the bottom.
8. Stir in the capers mixture and cook for about 8-10 minutes or until desired thickness, stirring occasionally.
9. Remove the skillet from heat and stir in heavy cream until smooth.
10. Again, place the skillet over medium heat and cook for about 1 minute.
11. Stir in the cooked chicken and cook for about 1 more minute.
12. Garnish with fresh parsley and serve hot.

## Nutrition Values (Per Serving)

- Calories: 633
- Net Carbs: 5.7g
- Carbohydrate: 8.6g
- Fiber: 2.9g
- Protein: 55g
- Fat: 442.3g
- Sugar: 1.8g
- Sodium: 1000mg

## Chicken in Creamy Spinach Sauce

(**Yields:** 4 servings / **Prep Time:** 15 minutes / **Cooking Time:** 15 minutes)

## Ingredients

- 2 tablespoons butter, divided
- 1 pound grass-fed chicken tenders
- Salt and ground black pepper, as required
- 2 garlic cloves, minced
- 1 jalapeño pepper, chopped
- 10 ounces frozen spinach, thawed
- ¼ cup Parmesan cheese, shredded

- ¼ cup heavy cream

## Instructions

1. Melt 1 tablespoon of butter in a large skillet over medium-high heat. Sprinkle the chicken tenders with salt and black pepper and cook for about 2-3 minutes per side.
2. Transfer the chicken tenders into a bowl.
3. Now, melt the remaining butter in the same skillet over medium-low heat and sauté the garlic and jalapeño pepper for about 1 minute.
4. Add the spinach and cook for about 1-2 minutes.
5. Add the cheese, cream, salt, and black pepper and stir to combine.
6. With the spoon, spread the spinach mixture evenly in the bottom of skillet.
7. Place the chicken tenders over spinach in a single layer.
8. Immediately, reduce the heat to low and cook, covered for about 5 minutes.
9. Serve hot.

## Nutrition Values (Per Serving)

- Calories: 333
- Net Carbs: 2g
- Carbohydrate: 3.7g
- Fiber: 1.7g
- Protein: 37.1g
- Fat: 18.6g
- Sugar: 0.5g
- Sodium: 321mg

---

# Chicken with Zucchini Pasta

**(Yields:** 6 servings / **Prep Time:** 20 minutes / **Total Cooking Time:** 18 minutes)

## Ingredients

- 1½ tablespoon butter
- 1½ pounds grass-fed boneless, skinless chicken thighs, cut into strips
- Salt, as required
- 4 ounces fresh semi-dried tomato strips in oil, chopped
- 3½ ounces jarred sun-dried tomatoes in oil, chopped
- 4 garlic cloves, crushed
- 1¼ cups heavy cream
- 1 cup Parmesan cheese, grated
- 1 teaspoon dried basil
- ½-1 teaspoon red pepper flakes
- 2 large zucchinis, spiralized with blade C

## Instructions

1. Melt the butter in a skillet over medium-high heat and cook the chicken strips with a little salt for about 4-5 minutes or until golden brown.
2. Add both dried tomatoes, and garlic and sauté for about 1-2 minutes.
3. Add the cream, and Parmesan cheese and stir to combine.

4. Immediately, reduce the heat to medium-low and simmer until the cheese is melted, stirring continuously.
5. Stir in the basil, salt, red pepper flakes, and zucchini noodles and simmer for about 5-8 minutes or until desired doneness.
6. Remove from the heat and serve.

## Nutrition Values (Per Serving)

- Calories: 329
- Net Carbs: 4.7g
- Carbohydrate: 6.4g
- Fiber: 1.7g
- Protein: 32.9g
- Fat: 19.7g
- Sugar: 2.9g
- Sodium: 225mg

(**Note:** If you can't find semi-dried tomato strips, then you can substitute it with extra jarred sun-dried tomatoes.)

---

## Creamy Chicken Casserole

(**Yields:** 4 servings / **Prep Time:** 15 minutes / **Cooking Time:** 1 hour 9 minutes)

## Ingredients

- 5 tablespoons unsalted butter, divided
- 2 small yellow onions, thinly sliced
- 3 garlic cloves, minced
- 1 teaspoon dried tarragon, crushed
- 8 ounces cream cheese, softened
- 1 cup homemade chicken broth, divided
- 2 tablespoons fresh lemon juice
- ½ cup heavy cream
- 1½ teaspoons Herbs de Provence
- Salt and ground black pepper, as required
- 4 (6-ounces) grass-fed chicken breasts

## Instructions

1. Preheat the oven to 350 degrees F. Grease a 13x9-inch baking dish with 1 tablespoon of butter.
2. In a skillet, melt 2 tablespoons of butter over medium heat and sauté the onion, garlic and tarragon for about 4-5 minutes.
3. Transfer the onion mixture onto a plate.
4. In the same skillet, melt the remaining butter over low heat and cook the cream cheese, ½ cup of broth and lemon juice for about 3-4 minutes, stirring continuously.
5. Stir in the cream, Herbs de Provence, salt, and black pepper and remove from heat.

6. Pour the remaining broth into prepared baking dish.
7. Arrange the chicken breasts into baking dish in a single layer and top evenly with the cream mixture.
8. Bake for about 45-60 minutes or until desired doneness of the chicken.
9. Serve hot.

## Nutrition Values (Per Serving)

- Calories: 729
- Net Carbs: 5.5g
- Carbohydrate: 6.3g
- Fiber: 0.8g
- Protein: 55.8g
- Fat: 52.8g
- Sugar: 2g
- Sodium: 655mg

---

# Chicken & Broccoli Bake

**(Yields:** 6 servings / **Prep Time:** 15 minutes / **Cooking Time:** 33 minutes)

## Ingredients

**For Chicken Mixture:**
- 2 tablespoons butter
- ¼ cup cooked bacon, crumbled
- ½ cup cheddar cheese, shredded
- 4 ounces cream cheese, softened
- ¼ cup heavy whipping cream
- ½ pack ranch seasoning mix
- 2/3 cup homemade chicken broth
- 1½ cups broccoli florets
- 2 cups cooked grass-fed chicken, shredded

**For Topping:**
- 2 cups cheddar cheese, shredded
- ½ cup cooked bacon, crumbled

## Instructions

1. Preheat the oven to 350 degrees F. Arrange an oven rack in the upper portion of oven.
2. For chicken mixture: in a large ovenproof skillet, melt the butter over low heat.
3. Add the bacon, cheddar cheese, cream cheese, heavy whipping cream, ranch seasoning, and broth and beat until well combined using a wire whisk.
4. Cook for about 5 minutes, stirring frequently.
5. Meanwhile, in a microwave-safe dish, place the broccoli and microwave until desired tenderness is achieved.
6. In the skillet of bacon mixture, add the chicken and broccoli and mix until well combined.
7. Remove the skillet from heat and top with cheddar cheese, followed by bacon.
8. Bake for about 25 minutes.
9. Now, set the oven to broiler.
10. Broil the chicken mixture for about 2-3 minutes or until the cheese is bubbly.
11. Remove from the oven and serve hot.

## Nutrition Values (Per Serving)

- Calories: 666
- Net Carbs: 3g
- Carbohydrate: 3.6g
- Fiber: 0.3g
- Protein: 46.5g
- Fat: 50.4g
- Sugar: 0.8g
- Sodium: 1999mg

**(Tip:** Make sure to use a small-sized broccoli floret.)

---

# Chicken & Veggie Bake

**(Yields:** 6 servings / **Prep Time:** 15 minutes / **Total Cooking Time:** 40 minutes)

## Ingredients

- 14 ounces grass-fed cooked chicken, shredded
- 9 ounces frozen spinach, thawed and squeezed
- 8 ounces fresh mushrooms, chopped
- 2 tablespoons butter
- 2 garlic cloves, minced
- 1 cup heavy cream
- 1 cup Parmesan cheese, grated
- ½ cup mascarpone cheese
- 1½ cups mozzarella cheese, shredded and divided
- Salt and ground black pepper, as required

## Instructions

1. Preheat the oven to 375 degrees F. Grease a casserole dish.
2. Place the shredded chicken, spinach and mushrooms into a large bowl and mix well.
3. Melt the butter in a pan over medium heat and sauté the garlic for about 20 seconds.
4. Add the heavy cream and stir to combine.
5. Add the Parmesan cheese, mascarpone cheese, salt, and black pepper and cook until cheeses are melted, stirring continuously.
6. Remove the pan of sauce from heat and stir the mixture well.
7. Add the sauce and ½ cup of mozzarella cheese into the bowl of chicken mixture and mix well.
8. In the bottom of prepared casserole dish, place the mixture evenly and sprinkle with the remaining mozzarella cheese.
9. Bake for about 25 minutes.
10. Now, increase the temperature of oven to 425 degrees F.
11. Bake for about 10 more minutes.
12. Remove the casserole dish from oven and let it cool slightly before serving.
13. Serve.

## Nutrition Values (Per Serving)

- Calories: 326
- Net Carbs: 3.3g
- Carbohydrate: 4.6g
- Fiber: 1.3g
- Protein: 31.8g
- Fat: 20.7g
- Sugar: 0.9g
- Sodium: 314mg

---

# Chicken Parmigiana

**(Yields:** 4 servings / **Prep Time:** 15 minutes / **Cooking Time:** 26 minutes)

## Ingredients

- 1 large organic egg, beaten
- ½ cup of superfine blanched almond flour
- ¼ cup Parmesan cheese, grated
- ½ teaspoon dried parsley
- ½ teaspoon paprika
- ½ teaspoon garlic powder
- Salt and ground black pepper, as required
- 4 (6-ounces) grass-fed skinless, boneless chicken breasts, pounded into ½-inch thickness
- ¼ cup olive oil
- 1½ cups marinara sauce
- 4 ounces mozzarella cheese, thinly sliced
- 2 tablespoons fresh parsley, chopped

## Instructions

1. Preheat the oven to 375 degrees F.
2. Add the beaten egg into a shallow dish.
3. Place the almond flour, Parmesan, parsley, spices, salt, and black pepper in another shallow dish and mix well.
4. Dip each chicken breast into the beaten egg and then, coat with the flour mixture.
5. Heat the oil in a deep skillet over medium-high heat and fry the chicken breasts for about 3 minutes per side.
6. With a slotted spoon, transfer the chicken breasts onto a paper towel-lined plate to drain.
7. In the bottom of a casserole dish, place about ½ cup of marinara sauce and spread evenly.
8. Arrange the chicken breasts over marinara sauce in a single layer.
9. Top with the remaining marinara sauce, followed by mozzarella cheese slices.
10. Bake for about 20 minutes or until done completely.
11. Remove from the oven and serve hot with the garnishing of fresh parsley.

## Nutrition Values (Per Serving)

- Calories: 542
- Net Carbs: 5.7g
- Carbohydrate: 9g
- Fiber: 3.3g
- Protein: 54.2g
- Fat: 33.2g
- Sugar: 3.8g
- Sodium: 609mg

---

# Chicken Cordon Bleu

**(Yields:** 4 servings / **Prep Time:** 20 minutes / **Total Cooking Time:** 24 minutes)

## Ingredients

- 4 (6-ounces) grass-fed boneless, skinless chicken breasts, thinly pounded
- 4 thin sugar-free ham slices
- 4 thin Swiss cheese slices
- ½ teaspoon paprika
- ½ teaspoons garlic powder
- Salt and ground black pepper, as required
- 1 tablespoon butter, melted
- ½ cup heavy cream
- 2 tablespoons fresh lemon juice
- 1 tablespoon Dijon mustard
- 2 tablespoons fresh parsley, finely chopped

## Instructions

1. Preheat the oven to 400 degrees F.
2. With a sharp knife, cut a pocket in the thickest part of each chicken breast, without cutting all the way through.
3. Place one ham slice into each chicken breast pocket, followed by 1 cheese slice.
4. Fold the chicken over the filling to close.
5. Season each stuffed chicken breast evenly with ¼ teaspoon of paprika, ¼ teaspoon of garlic powder, salt and black pepper.
6. Melt the butter in a cast iron skillet over medium-high heat and sear the chicken breasts for about 2-2½ minutes per side.
7. Remove from the heat and immediately, transfer the chicken breasts into a casserole dish.
8. Bake for about 10-15 minutes or until chicken is done completely.
9. Meanwhile, for the sauce: in a small pan, add the heavy cream, lemon juice and mustard over high heat and cook for 4-6 minutes, stirring frequently.
10. Stir in the remaining paprika, garlic powder, salt and black pepper and remove from heat.
11. Remove the casserole dish from oven and transfer the chicken breasts onto serving plates.
12. Top each chicken breast with sauce and serve with the garnishing of fresh parsley.

### Nutrition Values (Per Serving)

- Calories: 559
- Net Carbs: 3.2g
- Carbohydrate: 3.9g
- Fiber: 0.7g
- Protein: 62.1g
- Fat: 31.5g
- Sugar: 0.7g
- Sodium: 677mg

---

## Stuffed Chicken Thighs

**(Yields:** 6 servings / **Prep Time:** 15 minutes / **Cooking Time:** 21 minutes)

### Ingredients

- ¼ pound cooked bacon, chopped
- ½ cup Gruyere cheese, grated
- 1 cup fresh baby spinach, chopped
- 6 (6-8 ounces) boneless, skin-on chicken thighs, pounded into ½-inch thickness
- 2 teaspoons Italian seasoning
- 2 tablespoons unsalted butter
- Salt and ground black pepper, as required

### Instructions

1. Preheat the oven to 475 degrees F.
2. In a bowl, mix together the bacon, spinach and cheese.
3. Sprinkle each chicken thigh evenly with the Italian seasoning.
4. Arrange the chicken thighs onto a smooth surface, skin side down.
5. Place bacon mixture in the center of each chicken thigh.
6. Roll up each thigh to secure the filling.
7. Season each chicken thigh with salt and black pepper.
8. Melt the butter in a large cast iron skillet over high heat.
9. Place the chicken thighs, skin side up and cook for about 2 minutes.
10. Flip the chicken thighs and cook for about 2 minutes.
11. Adjust the heat to medium and cook for about 12 more minutes.
12. Flip the chicken thighs and transfer the skillet into the oven.
13. Bake for about 5 minutes.
14. Remove the skillet from oven and serve hot.

### Nutrition Values (Per Serving)

- Calories: 541
- Net Carbs: 0.6g
- Carbohydrate: 0.7g
- Fiber: 0.1g
- Protein: 40g
- Fat: 40.7g
- Sugar: 0.2g
- Sodium: 654mg

# Bacon Wrapped Chicken Breast

**(Yields:** 4 servings / **Prep Time:** 15 minutes / **Cooking Time:** 33 minutes)

## Ingredients

**For Chicken Marinade:**
- 3 tablespoons vinegar
- 3 tablespoons olive oil
- 2 tablespoons water
- 1 garlic clove, minced
- 1 teaspoon dried Italian seasoning
- ½ teaspoon dried rosemary
- Salt and ground black pepper, as required
- 4 (6-ounces) grass-fed skinless, boneless chicken breasts

**For Stuffing:**
- 16 fresh basil leaves
- 1 large fresh tomato, thinly sliced
- 4 provolone cheese slices
- 12 bacon slices
- ¼ cup Parmesan cheese, grated freshly

## Instructions

1. For marinade: add all the ingredients in a bowl except chicken breasts and mix until well combined.
2. Place 1 chicken breast onto a smooth surface.
3. Holding a sharp knife, parallel to work surface, slice the chicken breast horizontally, without cutting all the way through.
4. Repeat with the remaining chicken breasts.
5. Place breasts in the bowl of marinade and toss to coat well.
6. Refrigerate, covered for at least 30 minutes.
7. Preheat the oven to 500 degrees F. Grease a baking dish.
8. Remove the chicken breasts from bowl and arrange onto a smooth surface.
9. Place 4 basil leaves onto the bottom half of each chicken breast, followed by 2-3 tomato slices and 1 provolone cheese slice.
10. Now, fold the top half over filling.
11. Wrap each chicken breast with 3 bacon slices and secure with the toothpicks.
12. Arrange the chicken breasts into prepared baking dish in a single layer.
13. Bake for about 30 minutes, flipping once halfway through.
14. Remove from the oven and sprinkle each chicken breast with parmesan cheese.
15. Bake for about 2-3 more minutes.
16. Serve hot.

## Nutrition Values (Per Serving)

- Calories: 906
- Net Carbs: 3.5g
- Carbohydrate: 4.2g
- Fiber: 0.7g
- Protein: 79.9g
- Fat: 62g
- Sugar: 1.5g
- Sodium: 240mg

# Chicken Stuffed Avocado

**(Yields:** 8 servings / **Prep Time:** 15 minutes / **Cooking Time:** 10 minutes)

## Ingredients

- 4 avocados, halved and pitted
- 2 cups grass-fed cooked chicken, shredded
- 4 ounces cream cheese, softened
- ¼ cup tomatoes, chopped
- Salt and ground black pepper, as required
- ½ cup Parmesan cheese, shredded

## Instructions

1. Preheat the oven to 400 degrees F. Line a large baking sheet with a piece of foil.
2. With a scooper, scoop out the flesh from middle of each avocado half.
3. In a bowl, add the avocado flesh and mash slightly.
4. Add the chicken, cream cheese, tomatoes, salt, and black pepper and mix well.
5. Divide the chicken mixture evenly into avocado halves and sprinkle with Parmesan cheese.
6. Bake for about 8-10 minutes.
7. Remove from the oven and serve warm.

## Nutrition Values (Per Serving)

- Calories: 329
- Net Carbs: 2.6g
- Carbohydrate: 9.4g
- Fiber: 6.8g
- Protein: 15.1g
- Fat: 27g
- Sugar: 0.7g
- Sodium: 174mg

---

# Chicken Kabobs

**(Yields:** 4 servings / **Prep Time:** 15 minutes / **Cooking Time:** 8 minutes)

## Ingredients

- ¾ cup plain Greek yogurt
- 2 tablespoons olive oil
- 2 tablespoons fresh lemon juice
- 1 garlic clove, minced
- 2 teaspoons ground cumin
- ½ teaspoon ground coriander
- ¼ teaspoon cayenne pepper
- Salt and ground black pepper, as required
- 4 (6-ounces) grass-fed boneless, skinless chicken breasts, cut into 1-inch chunks

## Instructions

1. Place all the ingredients except chicken chunks into a large bowl and mix until well combined.
2. Add the chicken chunks and generously, coat with the yogurt mixture.
3. Refrigerate overnight.
4. Soak the wooden skewers in water for about 30 minutes.
5. Preheat the grill to medium-high heat. Grease the grill grate.
6. Thread the chicken chunks onto pre-soaked wooden skewers.
7. Arrange chicken skewers onto the grill and cook for about 3-4 minutes per side.
8. Serve hot.

## Nutrition Values (Per Serving)

- Calories: 423
- Net Carbs: 4g
- Carbohydrate: 4.2g
- Fiber: 0.2g
- Protein: 52.1g
- Fat: 20.5g
- Sugar: 3.4g
- Sodium: 221mg

(**Tip:** For more flavor, you can add fresh herbs and spices of your choice.)

---

# Creamy Ground Turkey

(**Yields:** 4 servings / **Prep Time:** 15 minutes / **Total Cooking Time:** 20 minutes)

## Ingredients

**For Spices Blend:**
- 1 teaspoon xanthan gum
- 1 teaspoon ground cumin
- 1 teaspoon ground coriander
- 1/8 teaspoon ground cloves
- 1/8 teaspoon ground cinnamon
- 1/8 teaspoon ground turmeric
- 1/8 teaspoon cayenne pepper
- 1 teaspoon salt
- 1/8 teaspoon freshly ground black pepper

**For Turkey:**
- 1¼ pounds ground turkey
- 1 small yellow onion, sliced
- 1 teaspoon fresh ginger, minced
- 1 teaspoon garlic, minced
- 1 medium tomato, chopped
- ½ cup water
- ½ cup unsweetened coconut milk
- 2 tablespoons fresh cilantro, chopped
- 2 tablespoons sour cream

## Instructions

1. For spice blend: add all the ingredients in a bowl and mix well. Set aside.
2. Heat a nonstick skillet over medium-high heat and cook the turkey, onion, ginger and garlic for about 5-6 minutes or until browned completely.
3. With a slotted spoon, discard any excess fat from the skillet.

4. Stir in the spice blend and cook for about 2 minutes, stirring frequently.
5. Stir in the remaining ingredients except cilantro and bring to a gentle boil.
6. Adjust the heat to medium-low and cook for about 10 minutes.
7. Stir in the chopped cilantro and remove from heat.
8. Serve immediately with the topping of sour cream..

## Nutrition Values (Per Serving)

- Calories: 380
- Net Carbs: 4.1g
- Carbohydrate: 6.6g
- Fiber: 2.5g
- Protein: 40.3g
- Fat: 24.2g
- Sugar: 2.6g
- Sodium: 763mg

---

# Turkey & Veggie Chili

**(Yields:** 8 servings / **Prep Time:** 15 minutes / **Cooking Time:** 3 hours 10 minutes**)**

## Ingredients

- 1 teaspoon olive oil
- 2 pounds ground turkey
- 1 yellow onion, chopped
- 1 green bell pepper, seeded and chopped
- ½ cup carrot, peeled and chopped
- 1 (4-ounces) can mushrooms, drained
- 2 garlic cloves, minced
- 1 (6-ounces) can sugar-free tomato paste
- 3 bay leaves
- 1 teaspoon dried thyme, crushed
- 2-3 tablespoons red chili powder
- 1 tablespoon ground cumin
- Salt and ground black pepper, as required
- 4 cups water
- ½ cup cheddar cheese, shredded

## Instructions

1. Heat the oil in a large nonstick pan over medium-high heat and cook the turkey for about 8-10 minutes.
2. Drain the excess grease from pan.
3. Stir in the remaining ingredients except cheddar and bring to a boil.
4. Adjust the heat to low and simmer, covered for about 3 hours.
5. Top with the cheddar cheese and serve hot.

## Nutrition Values (Per Serving)

- Calories: 296
- Net Carbs: 6.2g
- Carbohydrate: 8.6g
- Fiber: 2.4g
- Protein: 34.9g
- Fat: 16.1g
- Sugar: 4g
- Sodium: 236mg

# Turkey Casserole

**(Yields:** 6 servings / **Prep Time:** 15 minutes / **Cooking Time:** 1 hour)

## Ingredients

- 2 medium zucchinis, sliced
- 2 medium tomatoes, sliced
- Nonstick olive oil cooking spray
- ¾ pound ground turkey
- 1 large yellow onion, chopped
- 2 garlic cloves, minced
- 1 cup sugar-free tomato sauce
- ½ cup cheddar cheese, shredded
- 2 cups cottage cheese, shredded
- 1 organic egg yolk
- 1 tablespoon fresh rosemary, minced
- Salt and ground black pepper, as required

## Instructions

1. Preheat the oven to 500 degrees F. Grease a large roasting pan
2. Arrange the zucchini and tomato slices into prepared roasting pan and spray with some cooking spray.
3. Roast for about 10-12 minutes.
4. Remove from oven and set aside.
5. Now, preheat the oven to 350 degrees F.
6. Heat a nonstick skillet over medium-high heat and cook the turkey for about 4-5 minutes or until browned.
7. Add the onion and garlic and sauté for about 4-5 minutes.
8. Stir in the tomato sauce and cook for about 2-3 minutes.
9. Remove from heat and place the turkey mixture into a 13x9-inch shallow baking dish.
10. Add the remaining ingredients in a bowl and mix until well combined.
11. Place the roasted vegetables over turkey mixture, followed by the cheese mixture.
12. Bake for about 35 minutes.
13. Remove from the oven and set aside for about 5-10 minutes.
14. Cut into 6 equal-sized pieces and serve.

## Nutrition Values (Per Serving)

- Calories: 266
- Net Carbs: 8.3g
- Carbohydrate: 11g
- Fiber: 2.7g
- Protein: 30.7g
- Fat: 11.9g
- Sugar: 5.1g
- Sodium: 677mg

# Turkey Pizza

(**Yields:** 6 servings / **Prep Time:** 15 minutes / **Cooking Time:** 20½ minutes)

## Ingredients

**For Crust:**
- 2 cups mozzarella cheese
- 1 large organic egg
- 3 tablespoons cream cheese, softened
- ¾ cup almond flour
- 1 tablespoon psyllium husk
- 1 tablespoon Italian seasoning
- Salt and ground black pepper, as required
- 1 teaspoon butter, melted

**For Topping:**
- ½ cup sugar-free tomato sauce
- 16 pepperoni slices
- 1 cup mozzarella cheese, shredded
- ¼ teaspoon dried oregano, crushed

## Instructions

1. Preheat the oven to 400 degrees F.
2. For crust: in a microwave-safe bowl, add the mozzarella cheese and microwave on High for about 90 seconds or until melted completely.
3. In the bowl of mozzarella, add egg, and cream cheese and mix until well combined.
4. Add the remaining ingredients except butter and mix until well combined.
5. Coat the dough ball with melted butter and place onto a smooth surface.
6. With your hands, press the dough ball into a circle.
7. Arrange the crust onto a baking sheet and bake for about 10 minutes.
8. Carefully, flip the side and bake for about 2-4 more minutes.
9. Remove the crust from oven.
10. Spread the tomato sauce evenly over crust.
11. Arrange the pepperoni slices over tomato sauce and sprinkle with cheese.
12. Bake for about 3-5 minutes.
13. Remove the pizza from oven and sprinkle with dried oregano.
14. Cut into 6 equal-sized wedges and serve.

## Nutrition Values (Per Serving)

- Calories: 254
- Net Carbs: 4g
- Carbohydrate: 10.5g
- Fiber: 6.5g
- Protein: 12.1g
- Fat: 19.9g
- Sugar: 1.6g
- Sodium: 507mg

# Spicy Roasted Turkey

**(Yields:** 12 servings / **Prep Time:** 15 minutes / **Cooking Time:** 3½ hours)

## Ingredients

**For Marinade:**
- 1 (2-inch) piece fresh ginger, grated finely
- 3 large garlic cloves, crushed
- 1 green chili, finely chopped
- 1 teaspoon fresh lemon zest, grated finely
- 5 ounces plain Greek yogurt
- 3 tablespoons homemade tomato puree
- 2 tablespoons fresh lemon juice
- 1½ tablespoons garam masala
- 1 tablespoon ground cumin
- 2 teaspoons ground turmeric

**For Turkey:**
- 1 (9-pounds) whole turkey, giblets and neck removed
- Salt and ground black pepper, as required
- 1 large garlic clove, halved
- 1 lime, halved
- 1 lemon, halved

## Instructions

1. For marinade, add all the ingredients in a bowl and mix well.
2. With a fork, pierce the turkey completely.
3. In a large glass baking dish, place the turkey and rub evenly with the marinade mixture.
4. Refrigerate to marinate overnight.
5. Remove from refrigerator and set aside at room temperature for about 30 minutes before cooking.
6. Preheat the oven to 390 degrees F. Grease a large roasting pan.
7. Sprinkle the turkey with salt and black pepper and stuff the cavity with garlic, lime and lemon.
8. Arrange the turkey into prepared roasting pan and roast for about 30 minutes.
9. Now, reduce the temperature of oven to 350 degrees F.
10. Roast for about 3 hours.
11. Remove from oven and place the turkey onto a platter for about 15-20 minutes before carving.
12. With a sharp knife, cut the turkey into desired size pieces and serve.

## Nutrition Values (Per Serving)

- Calories: 595
- Net Carbs: 2g
- Carbohydrate: 2.3g
- Fiber: 0.3g
- Protein: 100.3g
- Fat: 17.3g
- Sugar: 1.2g
- Sodium: 262mg

**(Tip:** If the skin of turkey becomes brown during roasting, then cover with a piece of foil.)

# Creamy Turkey Breast

**(Yields:** 14 servings / **Prep Time:** 15 minutes / **Cooking Time:** 2½ hours)

## Ingredients

- 1 teaspoon onion powder
- ½ teaspoon garlic powder
- Salt and ground black pepper, as required
- 1 (7-pounds) bone-in turkey breast
- 1½ cups Italian dressing

## Instructions

1. Preheat the oven to 325 degrees F. Grease a 13x9-inch baking dish.
2. In a bowl, mix together the onion powder, garlic powder, salt, and black pepper.
3. Generously, rub the turkey breast with seasoning mixture.
4. Arrange the turkey breast into prepared baking dish and top evenly with the Italian dressing.
5. Bake for about 2-2½ hours, basting with the pan juices occasionally.
6. Remove from oven and place the turkey breast onto a platter for about 10-15 minutes before slicing.
7. With a sharp knife, cut the turkey breast into desired size slices and serve.

## Nutrition Values (Per Serving)

- Calories: 459
- Net Carbs: 2.8g
- Carbohydrate: 2.8g
- Fiber: 0g
- Protein: 48.7g
- Fat: 23.3g
- Sugar: 2.2g
- Sodium: 303mg

(**Note:** The recipe is called Creamy Turkey Breast because the Italian dressing has a creamy touch.)

---

# Grilled Turkey Breast

**(Yields:** 12 servings / **Prep Time:** 15 minutes / **Cooking Time:** 2 hours 32 minutes)

## Ingredients

- 1 cup homemade chicken broth
- 2/3 cup unsalted butter, melted
- 1 tablespoon fresh lemon juice
- ½ cup fresh basil leaves, chopped
- ¼ cup scallion, chopped
- 1 tablespoon garlic, chopped
- 2 teaspoons Erythritol
- Salt and ground black pepper, as required
- 1 (5-pounds) fresh turkey breast

## Instructions

1. Place all the ingredients except turkey breast into a large resealable bag.
2. Add the turkey breast and seal the bag tightly.
3. Shake the bag to coat well.
4. Refrigerate for at least 3 hours, flipping occasionally.
5. Preheat the grill to medium heat.
6. Remove the turkey breast from bag, reserving the remaining marinade.
7. Transfer the marinade into a pan over medium-high heat and cook for about 1-2 minutes.
8. Arrange turkey breast into a drip pan and place onto the grill.
9. Cover the grill and cook for about 2-2½ hours, flipping and basting with the cooked marinade occasionally.
10. Remove from grill and place the turkey breast onto a platter for about 10-15 minutes before slicing.
11. With a sharp knife, cut the turkey breast into desired size slices and serve.

## Nutrition Values (Per Serving)

- Calories: 297
- Net Carbs: 0.4g
- Carbohydrate: 0.5g
- Fiber: 0.1g
- Protein: 47.5g
- Fat: 11.1g
- Sugar: 0.2g
- Sodium: 427mg

---

## Bacon Wrapped Turkey Breast

**(Yields:** 2 servings / **Prep Time:** 10 minutes / **Cooking Time:** 1 hour)

## Ingredients

- ¾ pound turkey breast
- ½ teaspoon dried thyme
- ½ teaspoon dried rosemary
- ½ teaspoon dried, ground sage
- Salt and ground black pepper, as required
- 6 large bacon slices

## Instructions

1. Preheat the oven to 350 degrees F. Line a baking sheet with parchment paper.
2. Sprinkle the turkey breast with herb mixture, salt and black pepper.
3. Arrange the bacon slices onto a smooth surface in a row with the slices, pressing against each other.
4. Place turkey breast on top of the bacon slices.
5. Wrap the end pieces of bacon around the turkey breast first, followed by the middle pieces.

6. Arrange wrapped turkey breast onto the prepared baking sheet.
7. With a piece of foil, cover the turkey breast loosely and bake for about 50 minutes.
8. Remove the foil and bake for about 10 more minutes.
9. Remove from oven and place the turkey breast onto a platter for about 5-10 minutes before slicing.
10. With a sharp knife, cut the turkey breast into desired size slices and serve.

## Nutrition Values (Per Serving)

- Calories: 162
- Net Carbs: 0.8g
- Carbohydrate: 1g
- Fiber: 1.8g
- Protein: 11.3g
- Fat: 3.1g
- Sugar: 1.6g
- Sodium: 160mg

---

## Buttered Turkey Drumsticks

**(Yields:** 6 servings / **Prep Time:** 10 minutes / **Cooking Time:** 1 hour 40 minutes)

## Ingredients

- ¼ cup butter, softened
- 1 teaspoon dried thyme, crushed
- 1 teaspoon poultry seasoning
- Salt and ground black pepper, as required
- 6 bone-in turkey drumsticks, pat dried
- ½ cup homemade chicken broth

## Instructions

1. Preheat the oven to 350 degrees F.
2. Place the butter, thyme, seasoning, salt, and black pepper in a bowl and mix well.
3. Generously, coat the drumsticks with butter mixture.
4. Arrange drumsticks into a large roasting pan in a single layer.
5. Pour the broth over drumsticks.
6. Roast for about 90-100 minutes or until desired doneness.
7. Remove from the oven and place onto a platter for about 5-10 minutes before serving.
8. Serve.

## Nutrition Values (Per Serving)

- Calories: 232
- Net Carbs: 0.3g
- Carbohydrate: 0.4g
- Fiber: 0.1g
- Protein: 22.5g
- Fat: 15.8g
- Sugar: 0.1g
- Sodium: 230mg

# Feta Turkey Burgers

**(Yields:** 4 servings / **Prep Time:** 15 minutes / **Cooking Time:** 10 minutes)

## Ingredients

- 1 pound ground turkey
- 10 ounces feta cheese, crumbled
- 1 organic egg, beaten
- 10 ounces black olives, pitted and chopped
- 1 teaspoon garlic powder
- Salt and ground black pepper, as required
- 1 tablespoon unsalted butter
- 6 cups fresh baby spinach

## Instructions

1. Place the turkey, cheese, egg, olives, garlic powder, salt, and black pepper in a bowl and mix well.
2. Make 4 equal-sized patties from the mixture.
3. Arrange the patties onto a parchment paper lined baking sheet and refrigerate for about 15 minutes.
4. Melt the butter in a skillet over medium heat and cook the patties for about 3-5 minutes or until desired doneness.
5. Divide the spinach onto serving plates.
6. Top each plate with 1 patty and serve.

## Nutrition Values (Per Serving)

- Calories: 544
- Net Carbs: 6g
- Carbohydrate: 9.4g
- Fiber: 3.4g
- Protein: 44.5g
- Fat: 39.3g
- Sugar: 3.3g
- Sodium: 900mg

**(Tip:** Feta cheese can be replaced with goat cheese.)

# CHAPTER 6 | APPETIZERS & SNACKS

## Deviled Eggs

**(Yields:** 6 servings / **Prep Time:** 15 minutes / **Cooking Time:** 5 minutes)

### Ingredients

- 6 large organic eggs
- ¼ cup plain Greek yogurt
- Salt, as required
- 3 tablespoons scallions, finely chopped
- 1 tablespoon Dijon mustard
- Cayenne pepper, to taste
- 1 tablespoon chives, minced

### Instructions

1. In a pan of water, add the eggs and heat over high heat and bring to a boil.
2. Cover the pan and remove from heat.
3. Set the pan aside, covered for about 10-12 minutes.
4. Drain the eggs and set aside to cool completely.
5. Peel the eggs and with a sharp knife, slice them in half vertically.
6. Scoop out the yolks.
7. In a blender, add the egg yolks, yogurt, and salt and pulse until smooth.
8. Transfer the yogurt mixture into a bowl.
9. Add the scallion and mustard and stir to combine.
10. With a spoon, place the yogurt mixture evenly in each egg half.
11. Sprinkle with cayenne pepper and serve with the garnishing of chives.

### Nutrition Values (Per Serving)

- Calories: 82
- Net Carbs: 1.3g
- Carbohydrate: 1.5g
- Fiber: 0.2g
- Protein: 7.1g
- Fat: 5.2g
- Sugar: 1.2g
- Sodium: 134mg

---

## Cucumber Cups

**(Yields:** 4 servings / **Preparation Time:** 15 minutes)

### Ingredients

- 8 ounces cooked salmon, very finely chopped
- ¼ cup coconut cream
- 1 tablespoon shallots, minced
- 1 tablespoon fresh chives, minced
- ¼ teaspoon smoked paprika
- Salt and ground black pepper, as required
- 1 English cucumber, peeled and cut crosswise into ¾-inch thick slices

## Instructions

1. Add all the ingredients except cucumber in a bowl and mix until well combined.
2. With a teaspoon, scoop out the center of each cucumber slice slightly.
3. Place the salmon mixture over each cucumber slice.
4. Serve immediately.

## Nutrition Values (Per Serving)

- Calories: 123
- Net Carbs: 3.3g
- Carbohydrate: 4.1g
- Fiber: 0.8g
- Protein: 11.9g
- Fat: 7.2g
- Sugar: 1.8g
- Sodium: 68mg

---

# Zucchini Sticks

**(Yields:** 8 servings / **Prep Time:** 15 minutes / **Cooking Time:** 25 minutes)

## Ingredients

- 2 large zucchinis, cut into 3-inch sticks lengthwise
- Salt, as required
- 2 organic eggs
- ½ cup Parmesan cheese, grated
- ½ cup almonds, finely ground
- ½ teaspoon Italian herb seasoning

## Instructions

1. In a large colander, place the zucchini sticks and sprinkle with salt.
2. Set aside for about 1 hour to drain.
3. Preheat the oven to 425 degrees F. Line a baking sheet with parchment paper.
4. With your hands, squeeze the zucchini sticks to remove the excess liquid.
5. With a paper towel, pat dry the zucchini sticks.
6. Crack the eggs in a shallow bowl and beat them well.
7. Place the remaining ingredients in another bowl and mix until well combined.
8. Dip each zucchini sticks into the beaten eggs and then, evenly coat with the cheese mixture.
9. Arrange the zucchini sticks onto prepared baking sheet in a single layer.
10. Bake for 25 minutes, flipping once halfway through.
11. Remove from oven and transfer the zucchini sticks onto a platter.
12. Set aside to cool slightly.
13. Serve warm.

## Nutrition Values (Per Serving)

- Calories: 76
- Net Carbs: 1.7g
- Carbohydrate: 3g
- Fiber: 1.3g
- Protein: 5.2g
- Fat: 5.4g
- Sugar: 1.2g
- Sodium: 834mg

# Broccoli Tots

**(Yields:** 12 servings / **Prep Time:** 15 minutes / **Cooking Time:** 35 minutes)

## Ingredients

- 1 (16-ounces) package frozen chopped broccoli
- 3 large organic eggs
- ½ teaspoon dried oregano
- ½ teaspoon garlic powder
- 1/8 teaspoon cayenne pepper
- 1/8 teaspoon red pepper flakes, crushed
- Salt and ground black pepper, as required
- 1 cup sharp cheddar cheese, grated
- 1 cup almond flour

## Instructions

1. Preheat the oven to 400 degrees F. Line two baking sheets with lightly greased parchment paper.
2. Place the broccoli into a microwave-safe bowl and microwave, covered for about 5 minutes, stirring once halfway through.
3. Drain the broccoli well.
4. Place the eggs, oregano, garlic powder, cayenne pepper, red pepper flakes, salt and black pepper in a large bowl and beat until well combined.
5. Add the cooked broccoli, cheddar cheese and almond flour and mix until well combined.
6. With slightly wet hands, make 24 equal-sized patties from the mixture.
7. Arrange the patties onto prepared baking sheets in a single layer about 2-inch apart.
8. Lightly, spray each patty with the cooking spray.
9. Bake for about 15 minutes per side or until golden brown from both sides.
10. Remove from oven and transfer the broccoli patties onto a platter.
11. Set aside to cool slightly.
12. Serve warm.

## Nutrition Values (Per Serving)

- Calories: 123
- Net Carbs: 2.9g
- Carbohydrate: 4.9g
- Fiber: 2g
- Protein: 7g
- Fat: 9.2g
- Sugar: 1.2g
- Sodium: 100mg

# Cheesy Tomato Slices

**(Yields:** 10 servings / **Prep Time:** 15 minutes / **Cooking Time:** 5 minutes)

## Ingredients

- ½ cup mayonnaise
- ½ cup ricotta cheese, shredded
- ½ cup part-skim mozzarella cheese, shredded
- ½ cup Parmesan and Romano cheese blend, grated
- 1 teaspoon garlic, minced
- 1 tablespoon dried oregano, crushed
- Salt, as required
- 4 large tomatoes, cut each one in 5 slices

## Instructions

1. Preheat the broiler of oven on high. Arrange a rack about 3-inch from the heating element.
2. Place the mayonnaise, cheeses, garlic, oregano and salt in a bowl and mix until well combined and smooth.
3. Spread the cheese mixture evenly over each tomato slice.
4. Arrange the tomato slices onto broiler pan in a single layer.
5. Broil for about 3-5 minutes or until top becomes golden brown.
6. Remove from oven and transfer the tomato slices onto a platter.
7. Set aside to cool slightly.
8. Serve warm.

## Nutrition Values (Per Serving)

- Calories: 110
- Net Carbs: 5.6g
- Carbohydrate: 6.7g
- Fiber: 1.1g
- Protein: 5g
- Fat: 57.4g
- Sugar: 2.7g
- Sodium: 27mg

# Stuffed Tomatoes

**(Yields:** 12 servings / **Prep Time:** 20 minutes)

## Ingredients

- 24 cherry tomatoes
- 3 ounces cream cheese, softened
- 2 tablespoons mayonnaise
- ¼ cup cucumber, peeled and finely chopped
- 1 tablespoon scallion, finely chopped
- 2 teaspoons fresh dill, minced

## Instructions

1. Carefully, cut a thin slice from the top of each cherry tomato.
2. With the tip of a knife, carefully remove the pulp of each cherry tomato and discard it.
3. Arrange the tomatoes onto paper towels to drain, cut side down.
4. Place the cream cheese and mayonnaise in a bowl and beat until smooth.
5. Add the cucumber, scallion, and dill and stir to combine.
6. With a spoon, place the cheese mixture into each tomato.
7. Arrange the tomatoes onto a platter and refrigerate to chill slightly before serving.
8. Serve.

## Nutrition Values (Per Serving)

- Calories: 45
- Net Carbs: 2.4g
- Carbohydrate: 3.1g
- Fiber: 0.7g
- Protein: 1.3g
- Fat: 3.4g
- Sugar: 0.2g
- Sodium: 43mg

===

# Bacon Wrapped Asparagus

**(Yields:** 10 servings / **Prep Time:** 15 minutes / **Cooking Time:** 15 minutes)

## Ingredients

- 10 bacon slices, halved crosswise
- 6 ounces cream cheese, softened
- 1 (8-ounces) package frozen asparagus spears, thawed

## Instructions

1. Preheat the oven to 400 degrees F. Line two baking sheet with parchment paper.
2. Arrange the bacon slices onto a smooth surface.
3. Spread the cream cheese onto each bacon slice half.
4. Wrap each asparagus spear with 1 bacon slice half.
5. Arrange the wrapped asparagus onto prepared baking sheets in a single layer.
6. Bake for about 15 minutes.
7. Remove from the oven and serve warm.

## Nutrition Values (Per Serving)

- Calories: 215
- Net Carbs: 1.2g
- Carbohydrate: 1.7g
- Fiber: 0.5g
- Protein: 12.2g
- Fat: 17.7g
- Sugar: 0.5g
- Sodium: 698mg

# Mini Mushroom Pizzas

**(Yields:** 4 servings / **Prep Time:** 15 minutes / **Cooking Time:** 25 minutes)

## Ingredients

- 4 large Portobello mushrooms, stems removed
- ½ cup sugar-free marinara sauce
- ½ cup mozzarella cheese, shredded
- 1 gluten-free chorizo link, cut into thin slices

## Instructions

1. Preheat the oven to 375 degrees F. Line a large baking sheet with a lightly greased parchment paper.
2. With a spoon, scrape out the dark gills from mushrooms and discard the gills.
3. Arrange the mushrooms onto prepared baking sheet, stem side up.
4. Top each mushroom with the marinara sauce, followed by mozzarella and chorizo slices.
5. Bake for about 20-25 minutes or until the cheese is bubbly.
6. Remove from the oven and serve immediately.

## Nutrition Values (Per Serving)

- Calories: 116
- Net Carbs: 4.4g
- Carbohydrate: 5.9g
- Fiber: 1.5g
- Protein: 8.4g
- Fat: 7.3g
- Sugar: 1.5g
- Sodium: 294mg

---

# Jalapeño Poppers

**(Yields:** 12 servings / **Prep Time:** 15 minutes / **Cooking Time:** 25 minutes)

## Ingredients

- 10 ounces gluten-free pork sausage
- ½ cup cheddar cheese, shredded
- 24 fresh jalapeño peppers, stemmed and cut a slit along one side
- 12 bacon slices, halved lengthwise

## Instructions

1. Heat a medium nonstick skillet over medium heat and cook the sausage for about 8-10 minutes, breaking the links with spoon.
2. Drain the grease from skillet completely.
3. Remove the skillet from heat and let it cool completely.

4. Preheat the grill to medium heat. Grease the grill grate.
5. Add the cheddar cheese into cooled sausage and stir to combine.
6. Stuff each jalapeño pepper with the sausage mixture.
7. Wrap each jalapeño pepper with 1 halved bacon slice.
8. With a toothpick, secure each jalapeño pepper.
9. Place the jalapeño peppers onto grill and cook for about 15 minutes, flipping occasionally.
10. Remove from grill and transfer the jalapeño poppers onto a platter.
11. Set aside to cool slightly.
12. Serve warm.

## Nutrition Values (Per Serving)

- Calories: 268
- Net Carbs: 1.5g
- Carbohydrate: 2.6g
- Fiber: 1.1g
- Protein: 16.9g
- Fat: 20.8g
- Sugar: 1g
- Sodium: 1611mg

**(Note:** Remember to put on the rubber gloves before handling jalapeño peppers.)

---

## Mozzarella Sticks

**(Yields:** 4 servings / **Prep Time:** 10 minutes / **Cooking Time:** 6 minutes)

## Ingredients

- 8 bacon slices
- 1 cup olive oil
- 8 mozzarella cheese sticks, frozen overnight

## Instructions

1. Wrap a bacon slice around each cheese stick and secure with a toothpick.
2. In a cast iron skillet, heat the oil over medium heat and fry the mozzarella sticks in 2 batches for about 2-3 minutes or until golden brown from all sides.
3. With a slotted spoon, transfer the mozzarella sticks onto a paper towel-lined plate to drain.
4. Set aside to cool slightly.
5. Serve warm.

## Nutrition Values (Per Serving)

- Calories: 906
- Net Carbs: 2.8g
- Carbohydrate: 2.8g
- Fiber: 0g
- Protein: 37.5g
- Fat: 84.6g
- Sugar: 0g
- Sodium: 1600mg

# Cheese Balls

**(Yields:** 4 servings / **Prep Time:** 15 minutes / **Cooking Time:** 12 minutes)

## Ingredients

- 2 organic eggs
- ½ cup cheddar cheese, shredded
- ¼ cup Parmesan cheese, shredded
- ¼ cup mozzarella cheese, shredded
- ½ cup almond flour
- ½ teaspoon organic baking powder
- Ground black pepper, as required

## Instructions

1. Preheat the oven to 400 degrees F. Line a medium baking sheet with parchment paper.
2. Add the eggs into a large bowl and beat lightly.
3. Now, place the remaining ingredients and mix until well combined.
4. Make 8 equal-sized balls from the mixture.
5. Arrange the balls onto prepared baking sheet in a single layer.
6. Bake for about 10-12 minutes or until golden brown.
7. Remove from oven and transfer the cheese balls onto a platter.
8. Set aside to cool slightly.
9. Serve warm.

## Nutrition Values (Per Serving)

- Calories: 257
- Net Carbs: 2.9g
- Carbohydrate: 4.4g
- Fiber: 1.5g
- Protein: 17.4g
- Fat: 19.7g
- Sugar: 0.7g
- Sodium: 469mg

---

# Parmesan Chicken Wings

**(Yields:** 6 servings / **Prep Time:** 15 minutes / **Cooking Time:** 1 hour)

## Ingredients

- 3 pounds grass-fed chicken wings
- 1½ tablespoons organic baking powder
- Salt and ground black pepper, as required
- ¼ cup salted butter
- 4 garlic cloves, minced
- 2 teaspoons dried parsley
- Pinch of red pepper flakes
- ½ cup Parmesan cheese, grated
- 2 tablespoons fresh rosemary, chopped

## Instructions

1. Preheat the oven to 250 degrees F. Arrange an oven rack in the lower third of oven
2. Arrange a greased wire rack over a foil lined baking sheet.
3. Place the wings, baking powder, salt and black pepper in a ziplock bag.
4. Seal the bag and shake to coat well.
5. Now, arrange the wings onto prepared baking rack in a single layer.
6. Bake for about 30 minutes.
7. Now, increase the temperature of oven to 425 degrees F.
8. Then, arrange the baking sheet into the upper third of oven.
9. Bake for about 20-30 minutes or until crispy.
10. Meanwhile, place the butter, garlic, parsley and red pepper flakes in a bowl and mix well.
11. Remove from oven and transfer the wings into a large bowl.
12. Top the wings with butter mixture and parmesan and toss to coat well.
13. Garnish with fresh rosemary and serve immediately.

## Nutrition Values (Per Serving)

- Calories: 533
- Net Carbs: 2.6g
- Carbohydrate: 3.2g
- Fiber: 0.6g
- Protein: 68.6g
- Fat: 26.3g
- Sugar: 0g
- Sodium: 339mg

(**Note:** Make sure to pat dry the chicken wings completely before cooking.)

---

# Buffalo Chicken Bites

(**Yields:** 6 servings / **Prep Time:** 15 minutes / **Cooking Time:** 13 minutes)

## Ingredients

- 1 pound grass-fed ground chicken
- 1/3 cup almond flour
- ¼ cup Parmesan cheese, shredded
- 1 organic egg
- 1 tablespoon fresh chives, minced
- 1 garlic clove, minced
- ¼ teaspoon onion powder
- ½ cup hot sauce
- 2 tablespoons butter, melted
- ½ cup sugar-free ranch dressing

## Instructions

1. Preheat the oven to 500 degrees F. Grease one large baking sheet.
2. Place the ground chicken, almond flour, Parmesan cheese, egg, chives, garlic, and onion powder in a bowl and with your hands, mix until well combined.

3. Make 12 equal-sized balls from the mixture.
4. In the prepared baking sheet, arrange the meatballs in a single layer.
5. Bake for about 13 minutes or until the meatballs are done completely.
6. Meanwhile, add the hot sauce and butter in a large bowl and beat until well combined.
7. Remove the baking sheet of meatballs from oven and set aside for about 2-3 minutes.
8. Add meatballs into the bowl of hot sauce mixture and gently, toss to coat.
9. Transfer the meatballs onto a platter and drizzle with ranch dressing.
10. Serve immediately.

## Nutrition Values (Per Serving)

- Calories: 246
- Net Carbs: 2.4g
- Carbohydrate: 3.2g
- Fiber: 0.8g
- Protein: 25.6g
- Fat: 14.3g
- Sugar: 0.6g
- Sodium: 667mg

**(Note:** For an extra spicy, you can add cayenne pepper to the meatball mixture.)

---

# Mini Salmon Bites

**(Yields:** 10 servings / **Prep Time:** 15 minutes)

## Ingredients

- 8 ounces cream cheese, softened
- 4 ounces smoked salmon, chopped
- 2 medium scallions, thinly sliced
- Bagel seasoning, as required

## Instructions

1. In a bowl, add the cream cheese and beat until fluffy.
2. Add the smoked salmon, and scallions and beat until well combined.
3. Make bite-sized balls from the mixture and lightly coat with the bagel seasoning.
4. Arrange the balls onto 2 parchment-lined baking sheets and refrigerate for about 2-3 hours before serving.
5. Enjoy!

## Nutrition Values (Per Serving)

- Calories: 94
- Net Carbs: 0.7g
- Carbohydrate: 0.8g
- Fiber: 0.1g
- Protein: 3.8g
- Fat: 8.4g
- Sugar: 0.1g
- Sodium: 294mg

# Tilapia Strips

**(Yields:** 6 servings / **Prep Time:** 15 minutes / **Cooking Time:** 20 minutes)

## Ingredients

- 1 pound tilapia fillets, cut into strips
- 1 cup almond flour
- Salt and ground black pepper, as required
- 2 large organic eggs, beaten
- 1½ cups Parmesan cheese, shredded

## Instructions

1. Preheat the oven to 450 degrees F. Line one baking sheet with parchment paper.
2. Place the almond flour, salt, and black pepper in a shallow bowl and mix until well combined.
3. Place the eggs and a splash of water in a second bowl and beat well.
4. Add the Parmesan cheese in a third bowl.
5. Coat the tilapia strips with flour mixture, then dip into the beaten eggs and finally, coat with cheese.
6. Arrange the tilapia strips onto prepared baking sheet in a single layer.
7. Bake for about 18-20 minutes or until done completely.
8. Remove from oven and transfer the tilapia strips onto a platter.
9. Set aside to cool slightly.
10. Serve warm.

## Nutrition Values (Per Serving)

- Calories: 281
- Net Carbs: 2.8g
- Carbohydrate: 4.8g
- Fiber: 2g
- Protein: 27.7g
- Fat: 16.7g
- Sugar: 0.1g
- Sodium: 423mg

# Coconut Shrimp

**(Yields:** 4 servings / **Prep Time:** 20 minutes / **Cooking Time:** 20 minutes)

## Ingredients

- 2 tablespoons coconut flour
- Salt and ground black pepper, as required
- 2 large organic egg whites
- 1 cup unsweetened coconut flakes
- 1 pound shrimp, peeled and deveined

## Instructions

1. Preheat the oven to 400 degrees F. Grease one large baking sheet.
2. Place the coconut flour, salt and black pepper in a shallow bowl and mix until well combined.
3. Place the egg whites in a second bowl and beat until soft peaks form.
4. Add the coconut flakes in a third bowl.
5. Coat the shrimp with flour, then dip into the beaten egg whites and finally, coat with coconut flakes.
6. Arrange the shrimp onto prepared baking sheet in a single layer.
7. Bake for about 15 minutes.
8. Remove from oven and flip the shrimp.
9. Now, set the oven to broiler.
10. Broil the shrimp for about 3-5 minutes
11. Remove from oven and transfer the shrimp onto a platter.
12. Set aside to cool slightly.
13. Serve warm.

## Nutrition Values (Per Serving)

- Calories: 243
- Net Carbs: 5.3g
- Carbohydrate: 9.8g
- Fiber: 4.5g
- Protein: 29.6g
- Fat: 9g
- Sugar: 1.6g
- Sodium: 160mg

# Bacon Wrapped Scallops

**(Yields:** 9 servings / **Prep Time:** 20 minutes / **Cooking Time:** 15 minutes)

## Ingredients

- 18 sea scallops, side muscles removed
- 9 bacon slices, cut in half crosswise
- 2 tablespoons olive oil
- Salt and ground black pepper, as required

## Instructions

1. Preheat the oven to 425 degrees F. Line a baking sheet with parchment paper.
2. Wrap each scallop with 1 bacon slice half and secure with toothpicks.
3. Drizzle the scallops evenly with oil and then, season with salt and black pepper.
4. Arrange scallops onto the prepared baking sheet in a single layer.
5. Bake for about 12-15 minutes or until scallop is tender and opaque.
6. Remove from the oven and serve immediately.

### Nutrition Values (Per Serving)

- Calories: 236
- Net Carbs: 1.8g
- Carbohydrate: 1.8g
- Fiber: 0g
- Protein: 20.8g
- Fat: 15.7g
- Sugar: 0g
- Sodium: 782mg

---

## Avocado Salsa

**(Yields:** 3 servings / **Prep Time:** 15 minutes)

### Ingredients

- 1 ripe avocado, peeled, pitted and chopped
- ½ cup tomato, chopped
- 2 tablespoons onion, chopped
- 2 tablespoons fresh cilantro, minced
- 1 tablespoon olive oil
- 1 tablespoon fresh lime juice
- Salt and ground black pepper, as required

### Instructions

1. In a large serving bowl, add all the ingredients and gently, stir to combine.
2. With a plastic wrap, cover the bowl and refrigerate before serving.
3. Enjoy!

### Nutrition Values (Per Serving)

- Calories: 145
- Net Carbs: 2.4g
- Carbohydrate: 6.8g
- Fiber: 4.4g
- Protein: 1.5g
- Fat: 13.6g
- Sugar: 1.3g
- Sodium: 57mg

**(Note:** You can store this avocado salsa in the refrigerator for 2-3 days by putting into an airtight glass jar.)

---

## Chicken Popcorns

**(Yields:** 3 servings / **Prep Time:** 15 minutes / **Cooking Time:** 25 minutes)

### Ingredients

- ½ pound grass-fed chicken thigh, cut into bite-sized pieces
- 7 ounces unsweetened coconut milk
- 1 teaspoon ground turmeric
- Salt and ground black pepper, as required
- 2 tablespoons coconut flour
- 3 tablespoons desiccated coconut
- 1 tablespoon coconut oil, melted

### Instructions

1. Place the chicken, coconut milk, turmeric, salt and black pepper in a large bowl and mix well.
2. Cover the bowl and refrigerate to marinate overnight.
3. Preheat the oven to 390 degrees F.
4. Place the coconut flour and desiccated coconut in a shallow dish and mix well.
5. Coat the chicken pieces evenly with coconut mixture.
6. Arrange the chicken piece onto a baking sheet and drizzle with oil.
7. Bake for about 20-25 minutes.
8. Remove the baking sheet from oven and transfer the chicken popcorn onto a platter.
9. Set aside to cool slightly.
10. Serve warm.

### Nutrition Values (Per Serving)

- Calories: 375
- Net Carbs: 4g
- Carbohydrate: 8g
- Fiber: 4g
- Protein: 24.3g
- Fat: 28.1g
- Sugar: 2.5g
- Sodium: 127mg

---

## Chicken Nuggets

**(Yields:** 8 servings / **Prep Time:** 15 minutes / **Cooking Time:** 30 minutes)

### Ingredients

- 2 (8-ounces) grass-fed skinless, boneless chicken breasts, cut into 2x1-inch chunks
- 2 organic eggs
- 1 cup almond flour
- 1 teaspoon dried oregano, crushed
- ½ teaspoon onion powder
- ½ teaspoon garlic powder
- ½ teaspoon paprika
- Salt and ground black pepper, as required

### Instructions

1. Preheat the oven to 350 degrees F. Grease a baking sheet.
2. Crack the eggs in a shallow bowl and beat well.
3. Place the flour, oregano, spices, salt, and black pepper in another shallow bowl and mix until well combined.
4. Dip the chicken nuggets in beaten eggs and then, evenly coat with the flour mixture.

5. Arrange the chicken nuggets onto prepared baking sheet in a single layer.
6. Bake for about 30 minutes or until golden brown.
7. Remove from the oven and set aside to cool slightly.
8. Serve warm.

## Nutrition Values (Per Serving)

- Calories: 233
- Net Carbs: 3.1g
- Carbohydrate: 5.4g
- Fiber: 2.3g
- Protein: 23g
- Fat: 13.1g
- Sugar: 0.5g
- Sodium: 82mg

---

# Tuna Croquettes

**(Yields:** 4 servings / **Prep Time:** 15 minutes / **Total Cooking Time:** 16 minutes)

## Ingredients

- 24 ounces canned white tuna, drained
- ¼ cup mayonnaise
- 4 large organic eggs
- 2 tablespoons yellow onion, finely chopped
- 1 scallion, thinly sliced
- 4 garlic cloves, minced
- ¾ cup almond flour
- Salt and ground black pepper, as required
- ¼ cup olive oil

## Instructions

1. Place the tuna, mayonnaise, eggs, onion, scallion, garlic, almond flour, salt, and black pepper in a large bowl and mix until well combined.
2. Make 8 equal-sized oblong shaped patties from the mixture.
3. Heat the olive oil in a large skillet over medium-high heat and fry the croquettes in 2 batches for about 2-4 minutes per side.
4. With a slotted spoon, transfer the croquettes onto a paper towel-lined plate to drain completely.
5. Serve warm.

## Nutrition Values (Per Serving)

- Calories: 627
- Net Carbs: 4.1g
- Carbohydrate: 6.6g
- Fiber: 2.5g
- Protein: 51.3g
- Fat: 44.6g
- Sugar: 1.5g
- Sodium: 1300mg

# Brussels Sprout Chips

**(Yields:** 3 servings / **Prep Time:** 15 minutes / **Cooking Time:** 20 minutes)

## Ingredients

- ½ pound Brussels sprouts, thinly sliced
- 4 tablespoons Parmesan cheese, grated and divided
- 1 tablespoon olive oil
- 1 teaspoon garlic powder
- Salt and ground black pepper, as required

## Instructions

1. Preheat the oven to 400 degrees F. Lightly grease a large baking sheet.
2. Place the Brussels sprout slices, 2 tablespoons of Parmesan cheese, oil, garlic powder, salt, and black pepper in a large mixing bowl and toss to coat well.
3. Arrange the Brussels sprout slices onto prepared baking sheet in an even layer.
4. Bake for about 18-20 minutes, tossing once halfway through.
5. Remove from oven and transfer the Brussels sprout chips onto a platter.
6. Sprinkle with the remaining cheese and serve.

## Nutrition Values (Per Serving)

- Calories: 100
- Net Carbs: 4.7g
- Carbohydrate: 7.6g
- Fiber: 2.9g
- Protein: 5.4g
- Fat: 6.5g
- Sugar: 1.9g
- Sodium: 127mg

---

# Cauliflower Popcorns

**(Yields:** 6 servings / **Prep Time:** 15 minutes / **Cooking Time:** 30 minutes)

## Ingredients

- 4 cups large cauliflower florets
- 2 teaspoons butter, melted
- Salt, as required
- 3 tablespoons Parmesan cheese, shredded

## Instructions

1. Preheat the oven to 450 degrees F. Grease a roasting pan.
2. Add all the ingredients except Parmesan in a large bowl and toss to coat well.
3. Place the cauliflower florets into prepared roasting pan and spread in an even layer.

4. Roast for about 25-30 minutes.
5. Remove from oven and transfer the cauliflower popcorns onto a platter.
6. Sprinkle with the Parmesan cheese and serve.

## Nutrition Values (Per Serving)

- Calories: 38
- Net Carbs: 1.9g
- Carbohydrate: 3.6g
- Fiber: 1.7g
- Protein: 2.3g
- Fat: 2g
- Sugar: 1.6g
- Sodium: 99mg

---

# 3 Cheese Crackers

**(Yields:** 10 servings / **Prep Time:** 20 minutes / **Cooking Time:** 14 minutes)

## Ingredients

- 2 ounces cream cheese
- 1 cup Parmesan cheese, grated
- 1 cup Romano cheese, grated
- 1 cup almond flour
- 1 organic egg
- 1 teaspoon dried rosemary
- ¼ teaspoon Cajun seasoning
- Salt, as required

## Instructions

1. Preheat the oven to 450 degrees F and line a baking sheet with parchment paper.
2. Place the cream cheese, Parmesan cheese, Romano cheese, and almond flour in a microwave-safe bowl and microwave on High for about 1 minute, stirring once halfway through.
3. Remove from microwave and immediately, stir the mixture until well combined.
4. Set aside to cool for about 2-3 minutes.
5. In the same bowl of cheese mixture, add the egg, rosemary, seasoning, and salt and mix until a dough forms.
6. Arrange the dough between 2 large parchment papers and place onto a smooth surface.
7. With a lightly floured rolling pin, roll the dough into a thin layer.
8. Remove the upper parchment paper and with a knife, cut the dough into desired-sized crackers.
9. Carefully, arrange the crackers onto prepared baking sheet in a single layer about 1-inch apart.
10. Bake for about 6-7 minutes per side or until crispy.
11. Remove from oven and let the crackers cool completely before serving.
12. Enjoy!

### Nutrition Values (Per Serving)

- Calories: 151
- Net Carbs: 1.4g
- Carbohydrate: 2.7g
- Fiber: 1.3g
- Protein: 9.8g
- Fat: 12.4g
- Sugar: 0.4g
- Sodium: 281mg

## Cheese Bites

**(Yields:** 4 servings / **Prep Time:** 10 minutes / **Cooking Time:** 10 minutes)

### Ingredients

- 8 ounces provolone cheese, shredded
- ½ teaspoon paprika

### Instructions

1. Preheat the oven to 400 degrees F and line a baking sheet with parchment paper.
2. With a spoon, place the cheese in small heaps onto the prepared baking sheet, leaving about 1-inch apart.
3. Sprinkle evenly with paprika and bake for about 8-10 minutes.
4. Remove from oven and let the chips cool completely before serving.
5. Serve.

### Nutrition Values (Per Serving)

- Calories: 200
- Net Carbs: 1.3g
- Carbohydrate: 1.4g
- Fiber: 0.1g
- Protein: 14.5g
- Fat: 15.1g
- Sugar: 0.4g
- Sodium: 497mg

**(Note:** Feel free to use any cheese you like but preferably a kind that melts nicely and firms up like cheddar or Edam cheese.)

## Cheese Chips

**(Yields:** 8 servings / **Prep Time:** 15 minutes / **Cooking Time:** 15 minutes)

### Ingredients

- 3 tablespoons coconut flour
- ½ cup strong cheddar cheese, grated and divided
- ¼ cup Parmesan cheese, grated

- 2 tablespoons butter, melted
- 1 organic egg
- 1 teaspoon fresh thyme leaves, minced

## Instructions

1. Preheat the oven to 350 degrees F and line a baking sheet with parchment paper.
2. Place the coconut flour, ¼ cup of grated cheddar, Parmesan, butter, and egg and mix until well combined.
3. Set the mixture aside for about 3-5 minutes.
4. Make 8 equal-sized balls from the mixture.
5. Arrange the balls onto prepared baking sheet in a single layer about 2-inch apart.
6. With your hands, press each ball into a little flat disc.
7. Sprinkle each disc with the remaining cheddar, followed by thyme.
8. Bake for about 13-15 minutes or until the edges become golden brown.
9. Remove from the oven and let them cool completely before serving.
10. Serve.

## Nutrition Values (Per Serving)

- Calories: 94
- Net Carbs: 1.3g
- Carbohydrate: 3.2g
- Fiber: 1.9g
- Protein: 4.2g
- Fat: 7.1g
- Sugar: 0.5g
- Sodium: 105mg

---

# Cheddar Biscuits

(**Yields:** 6 servings / **Prep Time:** 15 minutes / **Cooking Time:** 15 minutes)

## Ingredients

- 1/3 cup coconut flour, sifted
- ¼ teaspoon organic baking powder
- Salt, as required
- 4 organic eggs
- ¼ cup butter, melted and cooled
- 1 cup cheddar cheese, shredded

## Instructions

1. Preheat the oven to 400 degrees F and line a large cookie sheet with a greased piece of foil.
2. In a large bowl, add the flour, baking powder, and salt and mix until well combined.
3. In another bowl, add the eggs and butter and beat until smooth.
4. Add egg mixture into the bowl of flour mixture and beat until well combined.
5. Fold in the cheddar cheese.

6. With a tablespoon, place the mixture onto prepared cookie sheet in a single layer and with your fingers, press slightly.
7. Bake for 15 minutes or until top becomes golden brown.
8. Remove the cookie sheet from oven and place onto a wire rack to cool for about 5 minutes.
9. Carefully, invert the biscuits onto wire rack to cool completely before serving.
10. Serve.

## Nutrition Values (Per Serving)

- Calories: 142
- Net Carbs: 0.5g
- Carbohydrate: 0.7g
- Fiber: 0.2g
- Protein: 6.4g
- Fat: 12.4g
- Sugar: 0.3g
- Sodium: 80mg

---

## Cinnamon Cookies

**(Yields:** 15 servings / **Prep Time:** 15 minutes / **Cooking Time:** 25 minutes)

## Ingredients

- 2 cups almond meal
- 1 teaspoon ground cinnamon
- 1 organic egg
- ½ cup salted butter, softened
- 1 teaspoon liquid stevia
- 1 teaspoon organic vanilla extract

## Instructions

1. Preheat the oven to 300 degrees F and grease a large cookie sheet.
2. Place all the ingredients in a large bowl and mix until well combined.
3. Make 15 equal-sized balls from the mixture.
4. Arrange the balls onto prepared baking sheet about 2-inch apart.
5. Bake for about 5 minutes.
6. Remove the cookies from oven and with a fork, press down each ball.
7. Bake or about another 18-20 minutes.
8. Remove from oven and place the cookie sheet onto a wire rack to cool for about 5 minutes.
9. Carefully, invert the cookies onto the wire rack to cool completely before serving.
10. Serve.

## Nutrition Values (Per Serving)

- Calories: 133
- Net Carbs: 1.2g
- Carbohydrate: 2.9g
- Fiber: 1.7g
- Protein: 3.1g
- Fat: 12.8g
- Sugar: 0.6g
- Sodium: 48mg

# Chocolate Fat Bombs

**(Yields:** 24 servings / **Prep Time:** 15 minutes)

## Ingredients

- 8 ounces cream cheese, softened
- ½ cup crunchy almond butter
- ½ cup unsalted butter, softened
- ½ cup golden monk fruit sweetener
- 2 ounces 70% dark chocolate, finely chopped

## Instructions

1. Add the cream cheese, almond butter, butter, and monk fruit sweetener in a bowl and with an electric mixer, mix until well blended.
2. Transfer the mixture into refrigerator for about 30 minutes.
3. Remove from refrigerator and fold in the chopped chocolate.
4. Make 24 equal-sized balls from the mixture.
5. Arrange the balls onto 2 parchment-lined baking sheets in a single layer and freeze for about 45 minutes before serving.
6. Serve.

## Nutrition Values (Per Serving)

- Calories: 169
- Net Carbs: 1.2g
- Carbohydrate: 1.9g
- Fiber: 0.7g
- Protein: 2.3g
- Fat: 17.2g
- Sugar: 0.1g
- Sodium: 112mg

---

# Mini Blueberry Bites

**(Yields:** 15 servings / **Prep Time:** 15 minutes)

## Ingredients

- 1 cup almond flour
- ½ cup pecans
- ½ cup fresh blueberries
- 4 ounces soft goat cheese
- 1 teaspoon organic vanilla extract
- ½ teaspoon stevia powder
- ¼ cup unsweetened coconut, shredded

## Instructions

1. Add the flour, pecans, blueberries, goat cheese, vanilla extract and stevia in a food processor and pulse until mixed completely.
2. Make 30 equal-sized balls from the mixture.

3. Coat the balls with shredded coconut.
4. Arrange the balls onto a parchment-lined baking sheet in a single layer and freeze for about 30-40 minutes before serving.
5. Serve.

## **Nutrition Values (Per Serving)**

- Calories: 114
- Net Carbs: 1.8g
- Carbohydrate: 3.3g
- Fiber: 1.5g
- Protein: 3.5g
- Fat: 9.9g
- Sugar: 1.1g
- Sodium: 26mg

---

# Chocolate Coconut Bars

(**Yields:** 9 servings / **Prep Time:** 20 minutes / **Total Cooking Time:** 8 minutes)

## **Ingredients**

- 1 cup coconut oil
- ½ can full-fat coconut milk
- ½ cup desiccated coconut
- 1 tablespoon coconut flour
- 1 teaspoon organic vanilla extract
- ¼ cup cacao powder
- ¼ cup coconut oil, melted
- 4-5 drops liquid stevia

## **Instructions**

1. For coconut filling: add 1 cup of coconut oil and coconut milk in a pan over low heat and cook for about 2-3 minutes, stirring continuously.
2. Add the desiccated coconut and stir to combine.
3. In the pan of coconut milk mixture, add the coconut flour, 1 tablespoon at a time and cook until the mixture resembles a porridge, beating continuously.
4. Remove the pan of mixture from heat and stir in vanilla extract.
5. Set the mixture aside to cool for about 10 minutes.
6. Place the coconut mixture evenly into a loaf pan and with the back of a spoon, press in 1-inch thick layer.
7. With a plastic wrap, cover the loaf pan and freeze for at least 5 hours or up to overnight.
8. Remove from the freezer and set aside at room temperature for about 20-25 minutes.
9. Place the cacao powder, melted coconut oil and stevia in a bowl and beat until well combined.
10. Cut the coconut filling into 9 equal-sized bars.
11. Dip each bar into the cacao powder mixture.

12. Arrange the bars onto a wax paper lined baking sheet and freeze until set before serving.
13. Serve.

## Nutrition Values (Per Serving)

- Calories: 341
- Net Carbs: 1.9g
- Carbohydrate: 4g
- Fiber: 2.1g
- Protein: 1.3g
- Fat: 37.7g
- Sugar: 1.2g
- Sodium: 8mg

---

# Walnut Bark

**(Yields:** 14 servings / **Prep Time:** 15 minutes / **Cooking Time:** 1 minute 40 secs)

## Ingredients

**For Bark:**
- ¼ cup coconut oil
- ¼ cup natural peanut butter
- 1 teaspoon organic vanilla extract
- 8 drops liquid vanilla stevia
- 1 cup walnuts, chopped
- Pinch of salt

**For Chocolate Drizzle:**
- 1 ounce 70% dark chocolate, chopped
- 1 teaspoon coconut oil

## Instructions

1. For bark: line 2 large plates with parchment paper.
2. Place the coconut oil and peanut butter in a microwave-safe bowl and microwave on High for about 30-40 seconds.
3. Remove the bowl from microwave and stir in the remaining ingredients.
4. Divide the mixture evenly onto each plate.
5. For drizzle: in a microwave-safe bowl, add the chocolate and coconut oil and microwave on High for about 1 minute.
6. Drizzle chocolate mixture over the bark and freeze for about 30 minutes or until set completely before serving.
7. Serve.

## Nutrition Values (Per Serving)

- Calories: 132
- Net Carbs: 1.1g
- Carbohydrate: 2.3g
- Fiber: 1.2g
- Protein: 3.9g
- Fat: 12.5g
- Sugar: 0.4g
- Sodium: 13mg

# Almond Brittles

**(Yields:** 8 servings / **Prep Time:** 15 minutes / **Total Cooking Time:** 10 minutes)

## Ingredients

- 1 cup almonds
- ¼ cup butter
- ½ cup Swerve
- 2 teaspoons organic vanilla extract
- ¼ teaspoon salt
- 1/8 teaspoon coarse salt

## Instructions

1. Line a 9x9-inch cake pan with parchment paper.
2. Add the butter, Swerve, vanilla and ¼ teaspoon of salt in an 8-inch nonstick skillet over medium heat and cook until well combined, stirring continuously.
3. Stir in the almonds and bring to a boil, stirring continuously.
4. Cook for about 2-3 minutes, stirring continuously.
5. Remove the skillet from heat and place mixture evenly into the prepared pan.
6. With the back of a spoon, stir to spread the almonds and sprinkle with salt.
7. Set aside for about 1 hour or until cooled completely.
8. Break into pieces and serve.

## Nutrition Values (Per Serving)

- Calories: 123
- Net Carbs: 1.2g
- Carbohydrate: 2.7g
- Fiber: 1.5g
- Protein: 2.6g
- Fat: 11.7g
- Sugar: 0.6g
- Sodium: 147mg

# CHAPTER 7 | FISH & SEAFOOD

## Grouper & Tomato Curry

**(Yields:** 6 servings / **Prep Time:** 15 minutes / **Cooking Time:** 15 minutes)

## Ingredients

- 1 tablespoon coconut oil
- 1 small yellow onion, chopped
- 2 garlic cloves, minced
- 1 teaspoon fresh ginger, minced
- 1 large tomato, peeled and chopped
- 1½ tablespoons red curry paste
- ¼ cup water
- 1¼ cups unsweetened coconut milk
- 1½ pounds skinless grouper fillets, cubed into 2-inch size
- Salt, as required
- 2 tablespoons fresh cilantro leaves, chopped

## Instructions

1. Melt the coconut oil in a large nonstick skillet over medium heat and sauté the onion, garlic and ginger for about 5 minutes.
2. Stir in the tomatoes and cook for about 2-3 minutes, crushing with the back of spoon.
3. Add the curry paste and sauté for about 2 minutes.
4. Add the water, and coconut milk and bring to a gentle boil.
5. Stir in the grouper cubes and cook for about 4-5 minutes.
6. Stir in the salt and cilantro leaves and serve hot.

## Nutrition Values (Per Serving)

- Calories: 307
- Net Carbs: 4.9g
- Carbohydrate: 6.7g
- Fiber: 1.8g
- Protein: 30g
- Fat: 18g
- Sugar: 3g
- Sodium: 97mg

**(Note:** Make sure to cut the fish into equal-sized cubes.)

# Salmon Curry

**(Yields:** 6 servings / **Prep Time:** 15 minutes / **Total Cooking Time:** 30 minutes)

## Ingredients

- 6 (4-ounces) salmon fillets
- 1 teaspoon ground turmeric, divided
- Salt, as required
- 3 tablespoons butter, divided
- 1 yellow onion, finely chopped
- 1 teaspoon garlic paste
- 1 teaspoon ginger paste
- 3-4 green chilies, halved
- 1 teaspoon red chili powder
- ½ teaspoon ground cumin
- ½ teaspoon ground cinnamon
- ¾ cup plain Greek yogurt, whipped
- ¾ cup water
- 3 tablespoons fresh cilantro, chopped

## Instructions

1. Season each salmon fillet with ½ teaspoon of turmeric and salt.
2. Melt 1 tablespoon of butter in a large skillet over medium heat and cook the salmon fillets for about 2 minutes per side.
3. Transfer the salmon onto a plate.
4. Now, melt remaining butter in the same skillet over medium heat and sauté the onion for about 4-5 minutes.
5. Add the garlic paste, ginger paste, green chilies, remaining turmeric, and spices and sauté for about 1 minute.
6. Adjust the heat to medium-low.
7. Slowly, add the yogurt and water, stirring continuously until smooth.
8. Cover the skillet and simmer for about 10-15 minutes or until desired doneness of the sauce.
9. Carefully, add the salmon fillets and simmer for about 5 more minutes.
10. Garnish with fresh cilantro and serve hot.

## Nutrition Values (Per Serving)

- Calories: 239
- Net Carbs: 4.4g
- Carbohydrate: 5.5g
- Fiber: 1.1g
- Protein: 24.3g
- Fat: 13.4g
- Sugar: 3.2g
- Sodium: 330mg

# Catfish Stew

**(Yields:** 10 servings / **Prep Time:** 15 minutes / **Total Cooking Time:** 50 minutes)

## Ingredients

- ¼ cup butter
- ½ cup yellow onion, chopped
- 1 cup celery stalk, chopped
- ½ cup green bell pepper, seeded and chopped
- 1 garlic clove, minced
- 4 cups water
- 4 chicken bouillon cubes
- 20 ounces okra, trimmed and chopped
- 2 (14-ounces) cans sugar-free diced tomatoes with liquid
- 2 bay leaves
- 1 teaspoon dried thyme, crushed
- 2 teaspoons red pepper flakes, crushed
- ¼ teaspoon hot pepper sauce
- Salt and ground black pepper, as required
- 32 ounces catfish fillets
- ½ cup fresh cilantro, chopped
- 1 cup sour cream

## Instructions

1. Melt the butter in a large skillet over medium heat and sauté the onion, celery, bell pepper and garlic for about 4-5 minutes.
2. Meanwhile, in a large soup pan, mix together the bouillon cubes, and water and bring to a boil over medium heat.
3. Transfer the onion mixture and remaining ingredients except catfish, cilantro and sour cream into the pan of boiling water and bring to a boil.
4. Lower the heat to low and cook, covered for about 30 minutes.
5. Stir in the catfish fillets and cook for about 10-15 minutes.
6. Stir in the cilantro and remove the pan of stew from heat.
7. Top with the sour cream and serve hot.

## Nutrition Values (Per Serving)

- Calories: 261
- Net Carbs: 7g
- Carbohydrate: 10.3g
- Fiber: 3.3g
- Protein: 17.2g
- Fat: 16.8g
- Sugar: 3.9g
- Sodium: 373mg

# Cream Cheese Salmon

**(Yields:** 2 servings / **Prep Time:** 10 minutes / **Cooking Time:** 20 minutes)

## Ingredients

- ¼ cup cream cheese, softened
- 2 tablespoons fresh chives, chopped
- 1 teaspoon garlic powder
- ¼ teaspoon cayenne pepper
- Salt and ground black pepper, as required
- 2 (4-ounces) salmon fillets

## Instructions

1. Preheat the oven to 350 degrees F and lightly, grease a small baking dish.
2. Add the cream cheese, chives, spices, salt and black pepper in a bowl and mix well.
3. Arrange the salmon fillets into prepared baking dish and top evenly with the cream cheese mixture.
4. Bake for about 15-20 minutes or until desired doneness of the salmon.
5. Remove the salmon fillets from oven and transfer onto the serving plates.
6. Serve hot.

## Nutrition Values (Per Serving)

- Calories: 257
- Net Carbs: 1.8g
- Carbohydrate: 2.1g
- Fiber: 0.3g
- Protein: 24.6g
- Fat: 17.2g
- Sugar: 0.5g
- Sodium: 214mg

---

# Cheesy Salmon

**(Yields:** 8 servings / **Prep Time:** 15 minutes / **Cooking Time:** 23 minutes)

## Ingredients

- 1/3 cup mayonnaise
- 2 garlic cloves, minced
- 2 tablespoons fresh lemon juice
- 1 tablespoon Dijon mustard
- 2 pounds salmon fillets
- 1 large yellow onion, thinly sliced
- Salt and ground black pepper, as required
- ¼ cup Parmesan cheese, finely shredded
- ½ cup Mozzarella cheese, finely shredded

## Instructions

1. Preheat the oven to 400 degrees F and line a rimmed baking sheet with a piece of foil.
2. In a small bowl, add the mayonnaise, lemon juice, mustard, and garlic and mix until well combined.

3. Arrange the salmon fillets onto prepared baking sheet and sprinkle with salt and black pepper.
4. Place the onion slices over salmon fillets, followed by mayonnaise mixture and cheeses.
5. Bake for about 15-18 minutes.
6. Now, set the oven to broiler.
7. Broil the salmon fillets for about 2-5 minutes.
8. Remove the salmon fillets from oven and transfer onto the serving plates.
9. Serve hot.

## Nutrition Values (Per Serving)

- Calories: 214
- Net Carbs: 4.2g
- Carbohydrate: 4.7g
- Fiber: 0.5g
- Protein: 23.9g
- Fat: 11.4g
- Sugar: 1.5g
- Sodium: 216mg

---

## Broiled Salmon

**(Yields:** 4 servings / **Prep Time:** 15 minutes / **Cooking Time:** 14 minutes)

## Ingredients

- ¼ cup plain Greek yogurt
- ½ teaspoon ground coriander
- ½ teaspoon ground turmeric
- ½ teaspoon ground ginger
- ¼ teaspoon cayenne pepper
- Salt and ground black pepper, as required
- 4 (6-ounces) skinless salmon fillets

## Instructions

1. Preheat the broiler of oven on high. Grease a broiler pan.
2. Add the yogurt, spices, salt and black pepper in a bowl and mix well.
3. Arrange the salmon fillets onto prepared broiler pan in a single layer.
4. Place the yogurt mixture evenly over each fillet.
5. Broil for about 12-14 minutes.
6. Remove the salmon fillets from oven and transfer onto the serving plates.
7. Serve hot.

## Nutrition Values (Per Serving)

- Calories: 241
- Net Carbs: 1.2g
- Carbohydrate: 1.3g
- Fiber: 0.1g
- Protein: 33.6g
- Fat: 3.11.4g
- Sugar: 1g
- Sodium: 123mg

# Nut Crusted Salmon

**(Yields:** 2 servings / **Prep Time:** 15 minutes / **Cooking Time:** 20 minutes)

## Ingredients

- 1 cup walnuts
- 1 tablespoon fresh dill, chopped
- 2 tablespoons fresh lemon rind, grated
- ½ teaspoon garlic salt
- Ground black pepper, as required
- 1 tablespoon butter, melted
- 3-4 tablespoons Dijon mustard
- 4 (3-ounces) salmon fillets
- 4 teaspoons fresh lemon juice

## Instructions

1. Preheat the oven to 350 degrees F and line a large baking sheet with parchment paper.
2. Place the walnuts in a food processor and pulse until chopped roughly.
3. Add the dill, lemon rind, garlic salt, black pepper, and butter and pulse until a crumbly mixture forms.
4. Place the salmon fillets onto prepared baking sheet in a single layer, skin-side down.
5. Coat the top of each salmon fillet with Dijon mustard.
6. Place the walnut mixture over each fillet and gently, press into the surface of salmon.
7. Bake for about 15-20 minutes.
8. Remove the salmon fillets from oven and transfer onto the serving plates.
9. Drizzle with the lemon juice and serve.

## Nutrition Values (Per Serving)

- Calories: 691
- Net Carbs: 4.6g
- Carbohydrate: 10.3g
- Fiber: 5.7g
- Protein: 49.8g
- Fat: 54.3g
- Sugar: 1.6g
- Sodium: 389mg

---

# Stuffed Salmon

**(Yields:** 4 servings / **Prep Time:** 20 minutes / **Cooking Time:** 16 minutes)

## Ingredients

**For Salmon:**

- 4 (6-ounces) skinless salmon fillets
- Salt and ground black pepper, as required
- 2 tablespoons fresh lemon juice
- 2 tablespoons olive oil, divided
- 1 tablespoon unsalted butter

**For Filling:**
- 4 ounces cream cheese, softened
- ¼ cup Parmesan cheese, grated finely
- 4 ounces frozen spinach thawed and squeezed
- 2 teaspoons garlic, minced
- Salt and ground black pepper, as required

## Instructions

1. Season each salmon fillet with salt and black pepper and then, drizzle with lemon juice and 1 tablespoon of oil.
2. Arrange the salmon fillets onto a smooth surface.
3. With a sharp knife, cut a pocket into each salmon fillet about ¾ of the way through, being careful not to cut all the way.
4. For the filling: in a bowl, add the cream cheese, Parmesan cheese, spinach, garlic, salt and black pepper and mix well.
5. Place about 1-2 tablespoons of spinach mixture into each salmon pocket and spread evenly.
6. Heat the remaining oil and butter in a skillet over medium-high heat and cook the salmon fillets for about 6-8 minutes per side.
7. Remove the salmon fillets from heat and transfer onto the serving plates.
8. Serve immediately.

## Nutrition Values (Per Serving)

- Calories: 438
- Net Carbs: 1.7g
- Carbohydrate: 2.4g
- Fiber: 0.7g
- Protein: 38.1g
- Fat: 31.7g
- Sugar: 0.4g
- Sodium: 285mg

---

# Bacon Wrapped Salmon

**(Yields:** 2 servings / **Prep Time:** 15 minutes / **Cooking Time:** 15 minutes)

## Ingredients

- 2 (6-ounces) salmon fillets
- 2 streaky bacon slices
- 4 tablespoons pesto

## Instructions

1. Preheat the oven to 350 degrees F and line a medium baking sheet with parchment paper.
2. Wrap each salmon fillet with 1 bacon slice and then, secure with a wooden skewer.
3. Place 2 tablespoons of pesto in the center of each salmon fillet.

4. Arrange the salmon fillets onto prepared baking sheet.
5. Bake for about 15 minutes.
6. Remove the salmon fillets from oven and transfer onto the serving plates.
7. Serve hot.

## **Nutrition Values (Per Serving)**

- Calories: 517
- Net Carbs: 1.9g
- Carbohydrate: 2.4g
- Fiber: 0.5g
- Protein: 46.7g
- Fat: 35.6g
- Sugar: 2g
- Sodium: 935mg

---

## Salmon Pie

**(Yields:** 5 servings / **Prep Time:** 20 minutes / **Cooking Time:** 50 minutes)

### **Ingredients**

**For Crust:**
- ¾ cup almond flour
- 4 tablespoons coconut flour
- 4 tablespoons sesame seeds
- 1 tablespoon psyllium husk powder
- 1 teaspoon organic baking powder
- Pinch of salt
- 1 organic egg
- 3 tablespoons olive oil
- 4 tablespoons water

**For Filling:**
- 8 ounces smoked salmon
- 4¼ ounces cream cheese, softened
- 1¼ cups cheddar cheese, shredded
- 1 cup mayonnaise
- 3 organic eggs
- 2 tablespoons fresh dill, finely chopped
- ½ teaspoon onion powder
- ¼ teaspoon ground black pepper

### **Instructions**

1. Preheat the oven to 350 degrees F and line a 10-inch spring form pan with parchment paper.
2. For crust: place all the ingredients in a food processor, fitted with a plastic pastry blade and pulse until a dough ball is formed.
3. Place the dough into prepared spring form pan and with your fingers, gently press in the bottom.
4. Bake for about 12-15 minutes or until lightly browned.
5. Remove the pie crust from oven and let it cool slightly.
6. Meanwhile, for the filling: add all the ingredients in a bowl and mix well.
7. Add the cheese mixture evenly into the pie crust.
8. Bake for about 35 minutes or until the pie is golden brown.

9. Remove the pie from oven and let it cool slightly.
10. Cut into 5 equal-sized slices and serve warm.

## Nutrition Values (Per Serving)

- Calories: 762
- Net Carbs: 5.6g
- Carbohydrate: 10.9g
- Fiber: 5.3g
- Protein: 24.8g
- Fat: 70g
- Sugar: 0.7g
- Sodium: 1500mg

---

## Cod & Vegetables Bake

**(Yields:** 4 servings / **Prep Time:** 15 minutes / **Cooking Time:** 20 minutes)

## Ingredients

- 1 teaspoon olive oil
- ½ cup yellow onion, minced
- 1 cup zucchini, chopped
- 1 garlic clove, minced
- 2 tablespoons fresh basil, chopped
- 2 cups fresh tomatoes, chopped
- Salt and ground black pepper, as required
- 4 (6-ounces) cod steaks
- 1/3 cup feta cheese, crumbled

## Instructions

1. Preheat the oven to 450 degrees F and grease a large shallow baking dish.
2. Heat the oil in a skillet over medium heat and sauté the onion, zucchini and garlic for about 4-5 minutes.
3. Stir in the basil, tomatoes, salt, and black pepper and immediately remove from the heat.
4. Place the cod steaks into prepared baking dish in a single layer and top with the tomato mixture.
5. Sprinkle evenly with the feta cheese.
6. Bake for about 15 minutes or until desired doneness.
7. Remove the cod mixture from oven and transfer onto the serving plates.
8. Serve hot.

## Nutrition Values (Per Serving)

- Calories: 250
- Net Carbs: 4.9g
- Carbohydrate: 6.6g
- Fiber: 1.7g
- Protein: 42g
- Fat: 5.5g
- Sugar: 4g
- Sodium: 319mg

# Cod in Butter Sauce

**(Yields:** 2 servings / **Prep Time:** 15 minutes / **Cooking Time:** 13 minutes)

## Ingredients

- 2 (6-ounces) cod fillets
- 1 teaspoon onion powder
- Salt and ground black pepper, as required
- 3 tablespoons butter, divided
- 2 garlic cloves, minced
- 1-2 lemon slices
- 2 teaspoons fresh dill weed

## Instructions

1. Season each cod fillet evenly with the onion powder, salt and black pepper.
2. Melt 1 tablespoon of butter in a medium skillet over high heat and cook the cod fillets for about 4-5 minutes per side.
3. Transfer the cod fillets onto a plate.
4. Meanwhile, in a frying pan, melt the remaining butter over low heat and sauté the garlic and lemon slices for about 40-60 seconds.
5. Stir in the cooked cod fillets and dill and cook, covered for about 1-2 minutes.
6. Remove the cod fillets from heat and transfer onto the serving plates.
7. Top with the pan sauce and serve immediately.

## Nutrition Values (Per Serving)

- Calories: 301
- Net Carbs: 2.2g
- Carbohydrate: 2.5g
- Fiber: 0.3g
- Protein: 31.1g
- Fat: 18.9g
- Sugar: 0.5g
- Sodium: 310mg

---

# Parmesan Halibut

**(Yields:** 2 servings / **Prep Time:** 10 minutes / **Cooking Time:** 24 minutes)

## Ingredients

- 2 (6-ounces) halibut fillets
- Salt and ground black pepper, as required
- 3 tablespoons sour cream
- ¼ teaspoon dill weed
- ¼ teaspoon garlic powder [when will this be used?]
- 2 tablespoons Parmesan cheese, grated
- 3 tablespoons scallions, chopped and divided

## Instructions

1. Preheat the oven to 375 degrees F and line a medium baking sheet with parchment paper.
2. Season each halibut fillet with salt and black pepper.
3. Add the sour cream, dill weed, and garlic powder in a bowl and mix until well combined.
4. Stir in the Parmesan cheese and 2 tablespoons of scallion.
5. Arrange the halibut fillets onto prepared baking sheet and top each evenly with Parmesan mixture.
6. Bake for about 24 minutes or until desired doneness.
7. Remove the halibut fillets from oven and transfer onto the serving plates.
8. Top with the remaining scallions and serve immediately.

## Nutrition Values (Per Serving)

- Calories: 250
- Net Carbs: 1.5g
- Carbohydrate: 1.8g
- Fiber: 0.3g
- Protein: 38.6g
- Fat: 9g
- Sugar: 0.3g
- Sodium: 221mg

---

# Garlicky Haddock

**(Yields:** 2 servings / **Prep Time:** 15 minutes / **Cooking Time:** 11 minutes)

## Ingredients

- 2 tablespoons butter
- 3 garlic cloves, minced
- 3 teaspoons fresh ginger, grated finely
- 2 (4-ounces) haddock fillets
- Salt and ground black pepper, as required

## Instructions

1. Melt the butter in a skillet over medium heat and sauté the garlic cloves and ginger for about 1 minute.
2. Add the haddock fillets, salt and black pepper and cook for about 3-5 minutes per side or until desired doneness.
3. Remove the haddock fillets from heat and transfer onto the serving plates.
4. Serve hot.

## Nutrition Values (Per Serving)

- Calories: 247
- Net Carbs: 3.4g
- Carbohydrate: 3.9g
- Fiber: 0.5g
- Protein: 28.3g
- Fat: 12.8g

- Sugar: 0.2g
- Sodium: 260mg

(**Tip:** You can adjust the ratio of garlic according to your taste.)

---

## Cheesy Tilapia

(**Yields:** 8 servings / **Prep Time:** 10 minutes / **Cooking Time:** 5 minutes)

### Ingredients

- 4 (4-ounces) tilapia fillets
- ½ cup Parmesan cheese, grated
- 3 tablespoons mayonnaise
- ¼ cup butter, softened
- 2 tablespoons fresh lemon juice
- ¼ teaspoon dried thyme, crushed
- ½ teaspoon garlic powder
- Salt and ground black pepper, as required

### Instructions

1. Preheat the broiler of oven on high. Grease a broiler pan.
2. Arrange the tilapia fillets onto prepared broiler pan in a single layer.
3. Broil for about 2-3 minutes.
4. Meanwhile, in a large bowl, add the remaining ingredients and mix well.
5. Remove the broiler pan from oven and top each tilapia fillet with the cheese mixture.
6. Broil for about 2 more minutes.
7. Remove the tilapia fillets from oven and transfer onto the serving plates.
8. Serve hot.

### Nutrition Values (Per Serving)

- Calories: 189
- Net Carbs: 1.8g
- Carbohydrate: 1.8g
- Fiber: 0g
- Protein: 23.5g
- Fat: 10.1g
- Sugar: 0g
- Sodium: 185mg

---

## Coconut Tilapia

(**Yields:** 5 servings / **Prep Time:** 15 minutes / **Cooking Time:** 6 minutes)

### Ingredients

- 2 tablespoons coconut oil
- 5 (5-ounces) tilapia fillets
- 3 garlic cloves, minced
- 2 tablespoons unsweetened coconut, shredded
- 1 tablespoon fresh ginger, minced
- 2 tablespoons low-sodium soy sauce
- 8 scallions, chopped

## Instructions

1. Melt the coconut oil in a large skillet over medium heat and cook the tilapia fillets for about 2 minutes.
2. Flip the side and stir in the garlic, coconut and ginger.
3. Cook for about 1 minute.
4. Add the soy sauce and cook for about 1 minute.
5. Add the scallions and cook for about 1-2 more minutes.
6. Remove the tilapia mixture from heat and transfer onto the serving plates.
7. Serve hot.

## Nutrition Values (Per Serving)

- Calories: 189
- Net Carbs: 3.1g
- Carbohydrate: 4.4g
- Fiber: 1.3g
- Protein: 27.7g
- Fat: 7.5g
- Sugar: 1.5g
- Sodium: 410mg

# Tuna Casserole

**(Yields:** 4 servings / **Prep Time:** 15 minutes / **Cooking Time:** 25 minutes)

## Ingredients

- 2 ounces butter
- 5 1/3 ounces celery stalks, chopped
- 1 yellow onion, chopped
- 1 green bell pepper, seeded and chopped
- 16 ounces canned tuna in olive oil, drained
- 4 ounces Parmesan cheese, shredded
- 1 cup mayonnaise
- 1 teaspoon chili flakes
- Salt and ground black pepper, as required

## Instructions

1. Preheat the oven to 400 degrees F and grease a large baking dish.
2. Melt the butter in a large frying pan and sauté the celery, onion and bell pepper or about 4-5 minutes.
3. Stir in the salt and black pepper and remove the pan from heat.
4. Place the tuna, Parmesan cheese, mayonnaise and chili flakes into the prepared baking dish and mix well.
5. Add the onion mixture and gently, stir to combine.
6. Bake for about 15-20 minutes or until the top becomes golden brown.
7. Remove the baking dish from oven and let it cool for about 5 minutes before serving.
8. Serve.

#### Nutrition Values (Per Serving)

- Calories: 790
- Net Carbs: 5.4g
- Carbohydrate: 7g
- Fiber: 1.6g
- Protein: 40.2g
- Fat: 66.9g
- Sugar: 3.2g
- Sodium: 832mg

---

## Grouper Casserole

**(Yields:** 5 servings / **Prep Time:** 15 minutes / **Cooking Time:** 27 minutes)

### Ingredients

- 2 tablespoons olive oil
- 15 ounces broccoli, chopped
- 6 scallions, chopped
- 2 tablespoons small capers
- Salt and ground black pepper, as required
- 1¼ cups heavy whipping cream
- 1 tablespoon dried parsley
- 1 tablespoon Dijon mustard
- 25 ounces grouper fillets, cut into bite-sized pieces
- 3 ounces chilled butter, chopped

### Instructions

1. Preheat the oven to 400 degrees F and grease a baking dish.
2. Heat the olive oil in a skillet over medium-high heat and cook the broccoli for about 5 minutes, until golden and soft.
3. Stir in the scallions, capers, salt and black pepper and cook for about 1-2 minutes.
4. Meanwhile, place the whipping cream, parsley and mustard in a bowl and mix well.
5. Remove the skillet of broccoli mixture from heat and place the broccoli mixture evenly into prepared baking dish.
6. Top with the grouper pieces and gently, press into the broccoli mixture.
7. Add the whipping cream mixture on top.
8. Evenly spread the butter pieces on top.
9. Bake for about 19-20 minutes or until desired doneness of the fish.
10. Remove the baking dish from oven and let it cool for about 5 minutes before serving.
11. Serve.

### Nutrition Values (Per Serving)

- Calories: 479
- Net Carbs: 5.3g
- Carbohydrate: 8.3g
- Fiber: 3g
- Protein: 38.9g
- Fat: 32.8g
- Sugar: 2g
- Sodium: 819mg

(**Note:** You can substitute the broccoli with Brussels sprouts.)

# Herbed Sardines

**(Yields:** 4 servings / **Prep Time:** 20 minutes / **Cooking Time:** 8 minutes)

## Ingredients

- 12 (2-ounces) fresh sardines, cleaned and scaled
- Salt and ground black pepper, as required
- 2 tablespoons olive oil
- ½ cup green olives, pitted and chopped
- 2 cups fresh parsley leaves, chopped
- 1 tablespoon fresh oregano, chopped
- 2 tablespoons capers, drained
- 2 garlic cloves, thinly sliced
- 2 Serrano peppers, seeded and minced
- 1 teaspoon lemon zest, grated finely

## Instructions

1. Preheat the oven to 400 degrees F.
2. Lightly, season the sardines with salt and black pepper.
3. Heat the olive oil in a large ovenproof skillet and cook the sardines for about 3 minutes.
4. Flip the sardines and stir in the remaining ingredients.
5. Immediately, transfer the skillet into oven and bake for about 5 minutes or until desired doneness of the fish.
6. Remove from oven and transfer the fish mixture onto serving plates.
7. Serve hot.

## Nutrition Values (Per Serving)

- Calories: 452
- Net Carbs: 2.4g
- Carbohydrate: 4.7g
- Fiber: 2.3g
- Protein: 43.3g
- Fat: 28.7g
- Sugar: 0.5g
- Sodium: 1180mg

---

# Lemony Trout

**(Yields:** 6 servings / **Prep Time:** 15 minutes / **Cooking Time:** 25 minutes)

## Ingredients

- 2 (1½-pounds) wild-caught trout, gutted and cleaned
- Salt and ground black pepper, as required
- 1 lemon, sliced
- 2 tablespoons fresh dill, minced
- 2 tablespoons butter, melted
- 2 tablespoons fresh lemon juice

## Instructions

1. Preheat the oven to 475 degrees F. Arrange a wire rack onto a foil-lined baking sheet.
2. Sprinkle the trout with salt and black pepper from inside and outside generously.
3. Fill the fish cavity with lemon slices and dill.
4. Place the trout onto prepared baking sheet and drizzle with the melted butter and lemon juice.
5. Bake for about 25 minutes.
6. Remove the baking sheet from oven and transfer the trout onto a serving platter.
7. Serve hot.

## Nutrition Values (Per Serving)

- Calories: 469
- Net Carbs: 0.7g
- Carbohydrate: 0.9g
- Fiber: 0.2g
- Protein: 60.7g
- Fat: 23.1g
- Sugar: 0.2g
- Sodium: 210mg

---

# Shrimp in Cream Sauce

**(Yields:** 3 servings / **Prep Time:** 20 minutes / **Cooking Time:** 15 minutes)

## Ingredients

**For Shrimp:**
- ½ ounce Parmigiano Reggiano, grated
- 1 large organic egg
- 2 tablespoons almond flour
- ½ teaspoon organic baking powder
- ¼ teaspoon curry powder
- 1 tablespoon water
- 12 medium shrimp, peeled and deveined
- 3 tablespoons unsalted butter

**For Creamy Sauce:**
- 2 tablespoons unsalted butter
- ½ of small yellow onion, chopped
- 1 garlic clove, finely chopped
- 2 Thai red chilies, sliced
- ½ teaspoon curry powder
- ½ cup heavy cream
- 1/3 cup cheddar cheese, grated
- Salt and ground black pepper, as required

## Instructions

1. For shrimp: add all the ingredients except shrimp and butter in a bowl and mix until well combined.
2. Add the shrimp and generously, coat with cheese mixture.

3. Melt the butter in a pan over medium heat and stir fry the shrimp for about 3-4 minutes or until golden brown from all sides.
4. With a slotted spoon, transfer the shrimp onto a plate.
5. For sauce: melt the butter in another pan over medium-low heat and sauté the onion for about 3-5 minutes.
6. Add the garlic, chilies, and curry powder and sauté for about 1 minute.
7. Reduce the heat to low and stir in heavy cream and cheddar until well combined.
8. Cook for about 1-2 minutes, stirring continuously.
9. Stir in the cooked shrimps, salt, and black pepper and cook for about 1-2 minutes.
10. Remove the pan of shrimp mixture from heat and transfer onto the serving plates.
11. Serve hot.

## **Nutrition Values (Per Serving)**

- Calories: 472
- Net Carbs: 4.4g
- Carbohydrate: 5.4g
- Fiber: 1g
- Protein: 29.1g
- Fat: 37.7g
- Sugar: 1.1g
- Sodium: 541mg

# **Shrimp with Zucchini**

(**Yields:** 4 servings / **Prep Time:** 15 minutes / **Total Cooking Time:** 7 minutes)

## **Ingredients**

- 2 tablespoons unsalted butter
- 1 large garlic clove, minced
- ¼ teaspoon red pepper flakes, crushed
- 1 pound medium shrimp, peeled and deveined
- Salt and ground black pepper, as required
- 1/3 cup homemade chicken broth
- 2 medium zucchinis, spiralized with blade C
- 1 tablespoon fresh parsley, finely chopped

## **Instructions**

1. Melt the butter in a large skillet over medium heat and sauté the garlic and red pepper flakes for about 1 minute.
2. Add the shrimp, salt, and black pepper and cook for about 1 minute per side.
3. Add the broth and zucchini noodles and cook for about 3-4 minutes, tossing occasionally.
4. Garnish with fresh parsley and serve hot.

### Nutrition Values (Per Serving)

- Calories: 206
- Net Carbs: 4.3g
- Carbohydrate: 5.5g
- Fiber: 1.2g
- Protein: 27.6g
- Fat: 8g
- Sugar: 1.8g
- Sodium: 392mg

---

## Shrimp with Asparagus

**(Yields:** 4 servings / **Prep Time:** 15 minutes / **Cooking Time:** 10 minutes)

### Ingredients

- 2 tablespoons butter
- 1 bunch asparagus, peeled and chopped
- 1 pound shrimp, peeled and deveined
- 4 garlic cloves, minced
- ½ teaspoon ground ginger
- 2 tablespoons fresh lemon juice
- 2/3 cup homemade chicken broth

### Instructions

1. Melt the butter in a large skillet over medium-high heat.
2. Add all the ingredients except broth and cook for about 2 minutes, without stirring.
3. Stir the mixture and cook for about 3-4 minutes, stirring occasionally.
4. Stir in the broth and cook for about 2-4 more minutes.
5. Serve hot.

### Nutrition Values (Per Serving)

- Calories: 222
- Net Carbs: 5.1g
- Carbohydrate: 7.6g
- Fiber: 2.5g
- Protein: 29.5g
- Fat: 8.1g
- Sugar: 2.5g
- Sodium: 449mg

---

## Shrimp & Tomato Bake

**(Yields:** 6 servings / **Prep Time:** 15 minutes / **Cooking Time:** 35 minutes)

### Ingredients

- ¼ cup unsalted butter
- 1 tablespoon garlic, minced
- 1½ pounds large shrimp, peeled and deveined
- ¾ teaspoon dried oregano, crushed
- ¼ teaspoon red pepper flakes, crushed
- ¼ cup fresh parsley, chopped

- Salt, as required
- ¾ cup homemade chicken broth
- 1 tablespoon fresh lemon juice
- 1 (14½-ounces) can sugar-free diced tomatoes, drained
- 4 ounces feta cheese, crumbled

## Instructions

1. Preheat the oven to 350 degrees F.
2. Melt the butter in a large skillet over medium-high heat and sauté the garlic for about 1 minute.
3. Add the shrimp, oregano, and red pepper flakes and cook for about 4-5 minutes.
4. Stir in the parsley, and salt and immediately transfer the mixture into a casserole dish.
5. In the same skillet, add the broth and lemon juice over medium heat and simmer for about 3-5 minutes or until liquid reduces to half.
6. Stir in the tomatoes and cook for about 2-4 minutes.
7. Pour the tomato mixture over shrimp mixture and top with the cheese.
8. Bake for about 15-20 minutes or until the top becomes golden brown.
9. Remove the casserole dish from oven and let it cool for about 5 minutes before serving.
10. Serve.

## Nutrition Values (Per Serving)

- Calories: 230
- Net Carbs: 5.4g
- Carbohydrate: 6.4g
- Fiber: 1g
- Protein: 25.5g
- Fat: 12.1g
- Sugar: 2.8g
- Sodium: 508mg

# Shrimp Curry

(**Yields:** 4 servings / **Prep Time:** 15 minutes / **Cooking Time:** 21 minutes)

## Ingredients

- 2 tablespoons coconut oil
- ½ of yellow onion, minced
- 2 garlic cloves, minced
- 1 teaspoon ground turmeric
- 1 teaspoon ground cumin
- 1 teaspoon paprika
- ½ teaspoon red chili powder
- 1 (14-ounces) can unsweetened coconut milk
- 1 (14½-ounces) can diced tomatoes with juice
- Salt, as required
- 1 pound shrimp, peeled and deveined
- 2 tablespoons fresh cilantro, chopped

## Instructions

1. Melt the coconut oil in a large skillet over medium heat and sauté the onion for about 5 minutes.
2. Add the garlic, and spices and sauté for about 1 minute.
3. Add the coconut milk, tomatoes, and salt and bring to a gentle boil.
4. Lower the heat to low and simmer for about 10 minutes, stirring occasionally.
5. Stir in the shrimp and cilantro and simmer for about 4-5 minutes.
6. Remove the skillet from heat and serve hot.

## Nutrition Values (Per Serving)

- Calories: 229
- Net Carbs: 6.9g
- Carbohydrate: 9g
- Fiber: 2.1g
- Protein: 27.3g
- Fat: 9.4g
- Sugar: 3.4g
- Sodium: 160mg

---

# Prawns in Creamy Mushroom Sauce

**(Yields:** 2 servings / **Prep Time:** 20 minutes / **Cooking Time:** 15 minutes)

## Ingredients

- 8 ounces prawns, peeled and deveined
- 1¼ cups fresh mushrooms, sliced
- 4 bacon slices, cut into 1-inch pieces
- 1½ cups heavy whipping cream
- 1 jalapeño pepper, chopped
- 1 teaspoon fresh thyme, chopped
- Salt and ground black pepper, as required

## Instructions

1. Heat a skillet over medium heat and cook the bacon for about 5 minutes, stirring frequently.
2. Add the mushrooms and cook for about 5-6 minutes, stirring frequently.
3. Add the prawns and stir to combine.
4. Increase the heat to high and stir fry for about 2 minutes
5. Add the cream, jalapeño pepper, thyme, salt, and black pepper and stir to combine.
6. Lower the heat to medium and cook for about 1 more minute.
7. Remove the skillet from heat and serve hot.

## Nutrition Values (Per Serving)

- Calories: 772
- Net Carbs: 6.4g
- Carbohydrate: 7.2g
- Fiber: 0.8g
- Protein: 50.7g
- Fat: 59.7g
- Sugar: 1.1g
- Sodium: 1730mg

# Pan Fried Squid

**(Yields:** 3 servings / **Prep Time:** 15 minutes / **Cooking Time:** 13 minutes)

## Ingredients

- 1 teaspoon olive oil
- ¼ of yellow onion, sliced
- 1 pound squid, cleaned and cut into rings
- ¼ teaspoon ground turmeric
- Salt, as required
- 1 organic egg, beaten

## Instructions

1. Heat the olive oil in a skillet over medium-high heat and sauté the onion for about 4-5 minutes.
2. Add the squid rings, turmeric, and salt and toss to coat well.
3. Now, lower the heat to medium-low and simmer for about 5 minutes.
4. Add the beaten egg and cook for about 2-3 minutes, stirring continuously.
5. Remove the skillet from heat and serve hot.

## Nutrition Values (Per Serving)

- Calories: 178
- Net Carbs: 5.6g
- Carbohydrate: 5.8g
- Fiber: 0.2g
- Protein: 25.5g
- Fat: 5.1g
- Sugar: 0.5g
- Sodium: 138mg

---

# Scallops with Broccoli

**(Yields:** 5 servings / **Prep Time:** 15 minutes / **Cooking Time:** 10 minutes)

## Ingredients

**For Scallops:**
- 1 tablespoon butter
- 2 garlic cloves, minced
- 1 pound fresh jumbo scallops, side muscles removed
- Salt and ground black pepper, as required
- 2 tablespoons fresh lemon juice
- 2 scallions (green part), thinly sliced

**For Broccoli:**
- 1¼ pounds small broccoli florets
- 2 tablespoons unsalted butter, melted

## Instructions

1. For broccoli: arrange a steamer basket in a pan of water over medium-high heat and bring to a boil.
2. Place the broccoli in steamer basket and steam, covered for about 4-5 minutes.

3. Meanwhile, in a large skillet, melt the butter over medium-high heat and sauté the garlic for about 1 minute.
4. Now, add the scallops and cook for about 2 minutes per side.
5. Stir in the salt, black pepper, and lemon juice and remove from heat.
6. Drain the broccoli and transfer onto a plate.
7. Drizzle the broccoli evenly with melted butter.
8. Divide the cooked broccoli onto serving plates and top with scallops.
9. Garnish with scallions and serve immediately.

## Nutrition Values (Per Serving)

- Calories: 266
- Net Carbs: 5.2g
- Carbohydrate: 8.3g
- Fiber: 3.1g
- Protein: 33.1g
- Fat: 8.6g
- Sugar: 2.2g
- Sodium: 430mg

---

# Buttered Scallops

**(Yields:** 3 servings / **Prep Time:** 15 minutes / **Cooking Time:** 7 minutes)

## Ingredients

- ¼ cup unsalted butter
- 2 tablespoons fresh rosemary, chopped
- 2 garlic cloves, minced
- 1 pound fresh scallops, side muscles removed
- Salt and ground black pepper, as required

## Instructions

1. Melt the butter in a medium skillet over medium-high heat and sauté the rosemary and garlic for about 1 minute.
2. Add the scallops and cook for about 2-3 minutes per side or until desired doneness.
3. Season with salt and black pepper and serve hot.

## Nutrition Values (Per Serving)

- Calories: 362
- Net Carbs: 1.1g
- Carbohydrate: 2.1g
- Fiber: 1g
- Protein: 40g
- Fat: 17.5g
- Sugar: 0g
- Sodium: 575mg

# Scallops in Garlic Sauce

**(Yields:** 4 servings / **Prep Time:** 15 minutes / **Cooking Time:** 13 minutes)

## Ingredients

- 1¼ pounds fresh scallops, side muscles removed
- Salt and ground black pepper, as required
- 4 tablespoons butter, divided
- 5 garlic cloves, chopped
- ¼ cup homemade chicken broth
- 1 cup heavy cream
- 1 tablespoon fresh lemon juice
- 2 tablespoons fresh parsley, chopped

## Instructions

1. Sprinkle the scallops evenly with salt and black pepper.
2. Melt 2 tablespoons of butter in a large pan over medium-high heat and cook the scallops for about 2-3 minutes per side.
3. Flip the scallops and cook for about 2 more minutes.
4. With a slotted spoon, transfer the scallops onto a plate.
5. Now, melt the remaining butter in the same pan over medium heat and sauté the garlic for about 1 minute.
6. Pour the broth and bring to a gentle boil.
7. Cook for about 2 minutes.
8. Stir in the cream and cook for about 1-2 minutes or until slightly thickened.
9. Stir in the cooked scallops and lemon juice and remove from heat.
10. Garnish with fresh parsley and serve hot.

## Nutrition Values (Per Serving)

- Calories: 417
- Net Carbs: 2.2g
- Carbohydrate: 2.4g
- Fiber: 0.2g
- Protein: 38.5g
- Fat: 24.5g
- Sugar: 0.2g
- Sodium: 570mg

---

# Steamed Clams

**(Yields:** 2 servings / **Prep Time:** 15 minutes / **Cooking Time:** 11 minutes)

## Ingredients

- 1 pound fresh clams, scrubbed
- 3 tablespoons unsalted butter
- 1 garlic clove, minced
- 10 fresh basil leaves
- ½ cup homemade chicken broth

### Instructions

1. Melt the butter in a large pan over medium heat and sauté the garlic for about 40-60 seconds
2. Add the basil leaves and chicken broth and stir to combine.
3. Increase the heat to medium-high and bring to a boil.
4. Stir in the clams and steam, covered tightly for about 7-8 minutes, shaking the pan twice.
5. Uncover and cook for about 1-2 more minutes.
6. Remove the pan from heat and discard any clams that have not opened.
7. Serve immediately.

### Nutrition Values (Per Serving)

- Calories: 435
- Net Carbs: 0.7g
- Carbohydrate: 0.8g
- Fiber: 0.1g
- Protein: 61g
- Fat: 21.7g
- Sugar: 0.2g
- Sodium: 570mg

---

## Lemony Crab Legs

**(Yields:** 2 servings / **Prep Time:** 15 minutes / **Cooking Time:** 5 minutes)

### Ingredients

- 1 pound king crab legs
- 4 tablespoons salted butter, melted
- 1 tablespoon fresh parsley, chopped
- 3 garlic cloves, minced
- 1 tablespoon fresh lemon juice

### Instructions

1. Preheat the oven to 375 degrees F.
2. With a sharp knife, cut the crab legs into halves to expose the flesh.
3. Add the butter, parsley, garlic and ½ tablespoon of lemon juice in a bowl and mix well.
4. In a small bowl, reserve about ¼ of the butter mixture.
5. Arrange the crab legs onto a baking sheet and drizzle with the remaining butter mixture.
6. Bake for about 5 minutes.
7. Remove the crab legs from oven and transfer onto the serving plates.
8. Drizzle with the reserved butter mixture and remaining lemon juice and serve immediately.

## Nutrition Values (Per Serving)

- Calories: 441
- Net Carbs: 1.5g
- Carbohydrate: 1.7g
- Fiber: 0.2g
- Protein: 44.2g
- Fat: 24.6g
- Sugar: 0.2g
- Sodium: 2580mg

## Seafood Stew

**(Yields:** 6 servings / **Prep Time:** 20 minutes / **Total Cooking Time:** 30 minutes)

## Ingredients

- 2 tablespoons butter
- 1 medium yellow onion, chopped
- 2 garlic cloves, minced
- 1 Serrano pepper, chopped
- ¼ teaspoon red pepper flakes, crushed
- ¾ pound fresh tomatoes, chopped
- 1½ cups homemade fish broth
- 1 pound red snapper fillets, cubed
- ½ pound shrimp, peeled and deveined
- ¼ pound fresh squid, cleaned and cut into rings
- ¼ pound bay scallops
- ¼ pound mussels
- 2 tablespoons fresh lime juice
- ½ cup fresh basil, chopped
- Salt and ground black pepper, as required
- 1/3 cup mayonnaise

## Instructions

1. Melt the butter in a large soup pan over medium heat and sauté the onion for about 5-6 minutes.
2. Add the garlic, Serrano pepper and red pepper flakes and sauté for about 1 minute.
3. Add the tomatoes, and broth and bring to a gentle simmer.
4. Lower the heat to low and cook for about 10 minutes.
5. Place the snapper fillets and cook for about 2 minutes.
6. Stir in the remaining seafood and cook for about 6-8 minutes.
7. Add the lime juice, basil, salt and black pepper and stir to combine.
8. Remove from heat and serve hot with the topping of mayonnaise.

## Nutrition Values (Per Serving)

- Calories: 336
- Net Carbs: 5.6g
- Carbohydrate: 6.8g
- Fiber: 1.2g
- Protein: 39.1g
- Fat: 16.1g
- Sugar: 2.3g
- Sodium: 430mg

# CHAPTER 8 | VEGGIES & SIDES

## Cabbage Casserole

(**Yields:** 3 servings / **Prep Time:** 15 minutes / **Cooking Time:** 30 minutes)

### Ingredients

- ½ head cabbage
- 2 scallions, chopped
- 4 tablespoons unsalted butter
- 2 ounces cream cheese, softened
- ¼ cup Parmesan cheese, grated
- ¼ cup fresh cream
- ½ teaspoon Dijon mustard
- 2 tablespoons fresh parsley, chopped
- Salt and ground black pepper, as required

### Instructions

1. Preheat the oven to 350 degrees F.
2. Cut the cabbage head in half, lengthwise. Then cut into 4 equal-sized wedges.
3. In a pan of boiling water, add the cabbage wedges and cook, covered for about 5 minutes.
4. Drain the cabbage well.
5. Now, arrange the cabbage wedges into a small baking dish.
6. Melt the butter in a small pan and sauté the scallions for about 5 minutes.
7. Add the remaining ingredients and stir to combine.
8. Remove from heat and immediately, place the cheese mixture over cabbage wedges.
9. Bake for about 20 minutes.
10. Remove the baking dish of cabbage mixture from oven and let it cool for about 5 minutes before serving.
11. Cut into 3 equal-sized portions and serve.

### Nutrition Values (Per Serving)

- Calories: 273
- Net Carbs: 5.6g
- Carbohydrate: 9g
- Fiber: 3.4g
- Protein: 6.2g
- Fat: 24.8g
- Sugar: 4.5g
- Sodium: 313mg

# Yellow Squash Casserole

**(Yields:** 8 servings / **Prep Time:** 15 minutes / **Cooking Time:** 55 minutes)

## Ingredients

- 2 tablespoons olive oil
- 1 small yellow onion, chopped
- 3 summer squashes, sliced
- 4 organic eggs, beaten
- 3 cups cheddar cheese, shredded and divided
- 2 tablespoons unsweetened almond milk
- 2-3 tablespoons almond flour
- 2 tablespoons Erythritol
- Salt and ground black pepper, as required
- 1/3 cup unsalted butter, melted

## Instructions

1. Preheat the oven to 375 degrees F.
2. Heat the oil in a large skillet over medium heat and cook the onion and squash for about 8-10 minutes, stirring occasionally.
3. Remove from the heat.
4. Place the eggs, 1 cup of cheddar cheese, almond milk, almond flour, Erythritol, salt and black pepper in a large bowl and mix until well combined.
5. Add the squash mixture, and butter and stir to combine.
6. Transfer the mixture into a large casserole dish and sprinkle with the remaining cheddar cheese.
7. Bake for about 35-45 minutes.
8. Remove the casserole dish from oven and set aside for about 5-10 minutes before serving.
9. Cut into 8 equal-sized portions and serve.

## Nutrition Values (Per Serving)

- Calories: 326
- Net Carbs: 3.2g
- Carbohydrate: 4.4g
- Fiber: 1.2g
- Protein: 14.8g
- Fat: 28.4g
- Sugar: 2g
- Sodium: 379mg

# Cauliflower Casserole

**(Yields:** 4 servings / **Prep Time:** 15 minutes / **Cooking Time:** 35 minutes)

## Ingredients

- 1 large head cauliflower, cut into florets
- 2 tablespoons butter
- 2 ounces cream cheese, softened
- 1¼ cups sharp cheddar cheese, shredded and divided
- 1 cup heavy cream

- Salt and ground black pepper, as required
- ¼ cup scallion, chopped and divided

## Instructions

1. Preheat the oven to 350 degrees F.
2. In a large pan of boiling water, add the cauliflower florets and cook for about 2 minutes.
3. Drain the cauliflower and set aside.
4. For the cheese sauce: in a medium pan, add butter over medium-low heat and cook until just melted.
5. Add the cream cheese, 1 cup of cheddar cheese, heavy cream, salt, and black pepper and cook for about 1-2 minutes until melted and smooth, stirring continuously.
6. Remove from the heat and set aside to cool slightly.
7. In a baking dish, place the cauliflower florets, cheese sauce, and 3 tablespoons of scallion and stir to combine well.
8. Sprinkle with the remaining cheddar cheese and scallion.
9. Bake for about 30 minutes.
10. Remove the casserole dish from oven and set aside for about 5-10 minutes before serving.
11. Cut into 4 equal-sized portions and serve.

## Nutrition Values (Per Serving)

- Calories: 365
- Net Carbs: 3.8g
- Carbohydrate: 5.6g
- Fiber: 1.8g
- Protein: 12g
- Fat: 33.6g
- Sugar: 3g
- Sodium: 373mg

# Broccoli Casserole

**(Yields:** 6 servings / **Prep Time:** 15 minutes / **Cooking Time:** 12 minutes)

## Ingredients

- 20 ounces fresh broccoli florets
- 2 tablespoons water
- 8 ounces cream cheese, room temperature
- 1 cup cheddar cheese, grated
- ¼ cup mayonnaise
- 1 teaspoon garlic powder
- Salt and ground black pepper, as required
- ¼ cup Parmesan cheese, grated

## Instructions

1. Preheat the oven to 350 degrees F.
2. Add the broccoli and water in a large microwave-safe bowl.

3. With a plastic wrap, cover the bowl tightly and microwave for about 2 minutes.
4. Remove from the microwave and set aside, covered for about 2 minutes.
5. Place the cream cheese, cheddar cheese, mayonnaise, garlic powder, salt, and black pepper in a large bowl and mix well.
6. Add the broccoli and mix until well combined.
7. In an 8x8-inch baking dish, place the broccoli mixture and sprinkle evenly with the Parmesan cheese.
8. Bake for about 10 minutes.
9. Remove the casserole dish from oven and set aside for about 5-10 minutes before serving.
10. Cut into 6 equal-sized portions and serve.

## **Nutrition Values (Per Serving)**

- Calories: 314
- Net Carbs: 5.4g
- Carbohydrate: 7.9g
- Fiber: 2.5g
- Protein: 11.6g
- Fat: 27.2g
- Sugar: 1.9g
- Sodium: 376mg

---

# **Eggplant Lasagna**

(**Yields:** 12 servings / **Prep Time:** 20 minutes / **Cooking Time:** 56 minutes)

## **Ingredients**

- 2 large eggplants, cut into 1/8-inch thick slices lengthwise
- Salt, as required
- 1 large organic egg
- 15 ounces part-skim ricotta
- ½ cup plus 2 tablespoons Parmesan cheese, grated and divided
- 4 cups sugar-free tomato sauce
- 16 ounces part-skim mozzarella cheese, shredded
- 2 tablespoons fresh parsley, chopped

## **Instructions**

1. Preheat the oven to 375 degrees F.
2. Arrange the eggplant slices onto a smooth surface in a single layer and sprinkle with salt.
3. Set aside for about 10 minutes.
4. With a paper towel, pat dry the eggplant slices to remove the excess moisture and salt.
5. Heat a greased grill pan over medium heat and cook the eggplant slices for about 3 minutes per side.
6. Remove the eggplant slices from grill pan and set aside.

7. In a medium bowl, place the egg, ricotta cheese and ½ cup of Parmesan cheese and mix well.
8. In the bottom of a 9x12-inch casserole dish, evenly spread some tomato sauce.
9. Place 5-6 eggplant slices on top of the sauce.
10. Spread some of the cheese mixture over eggplant slices and top with some of the mozzarella cheese.
11. Repeat the layers and sprinkle with the remaining Parmesan cheese.
12. Cover the casserole dish and bake for about 40 minutes.
13. Uncover the baking dish and bake for about 10 more minutes.
14. Remove the baking dish from oven and set aside for about 5-10 minutes before serving.
15. Cut into 12 equal-sized portions and serve with the garnishing of fresh parsley.

## Nutrition Values (Per Serving)

- Calories: 200
- Net Carbs: 6.3g
- Carbohydrate: 8g
- Fiber: 1.7g
- Protein: 18.2g
- Fat: 11g
- Sugar: 4.1g
- Sodium: 753mg

## Cheese & Olives Pizza

**(Yields:** 4 servings / **Prep Time:** 20 minutes / **Cooking Time:** 42 minutes)

## Ingredients

**For Crust:**
- 1 small head cauliflower, cut into florets
- 2 large organic eggs, beaten lightly
- ½ teaspoon dried oregano
- ½ teaspoon garlic powder
- Ground black pepper, as required

**For Topping:**
- ½ cup sugar-free pizza sauce
- ¾ cup mozzarella cheese, shredded
- ¼ cup black olives, pitted and sliced
- 2 tablespoons Parmesan cheese, grated

## Instructions

1. Preheat the oven to 400 degrees F and line a baking sheet with a lightly greased parchment paper.
2. Add the cauliflower in a food processor and pulse until rice like texture is formed.
3. In a bowl, add the cauliflower rice, eggs, oregano, garlic powder, and black pepper and mix until well combined.
4. Place the cauliflower mixture in the center of prepared baking sheet and with a spatula, press into a 13-inch thin circle.

5. Bake for about 40 minutes or until golden-brown.
6. Remove the baking sheet from oven.
7. Now, set the oven to broiler on high.
8. Place the pizza sauce on top of pizza crust and with a spatula, spread evenly and sprinkle with olives, followed by the cheeses.
9. Broil for about 1-2 minutes or until the cheese is bubbly and browned.
10. Remove from oven and with a pizza cutter, cut the pizza into equal-sized triangles.
11. Serve hot.

## Nutrition Values (Per Serving)

- Calories: 119
- Net Carbs: 5.2g
- Carbohydrate: 8.6g
- Fiber: 3.4g
- Protein: 8.3g
- Fat: 6.6g
- Sugar: 3.7g
- Sodium: 297mg

---

# Zucchini Pizza

**(Yields:** 4 servings / **Prep Time:** 20 minutes / **Total Cooking Time:** 42 minutes)

## Ingredients

**For Sauce:**
- 1 tablespoon olive oil, divided
- 2 large garlic cloves, minced
- 1 (14½-ounces) can petite diced tomatoes, drained
- ½ teaspoon Italian seasoning
- Salt and ground black pepper, as required

**For Crust:**
- 4 cups zucchini, grated and chopped
- 5 tablespoons almond meal
- ½ cup mozzarella cheese, grated finely
- 3 tablespoons Parmesan cheese, grated finely
- 1 organic egg, beaten
- 1 teaspoon dried oregano, crushed
- ½ teaspoon garlic powder
- Pinch of salt

**For Topping:**
- 3-ounces part-skim fresh mozzarella cheese, cut into chunks
- 10-15 large fresh basil leaves

## Instructions

1. For sauce: in a small frying pan, heat ½ tablespoon of oil over medium heat and sauté the garlic for about 30 seconds.
2. Add the tomatoes, and Italian seasoning and stir to combine.
3. Now, lower the heat to very low heat and simmer until the sauce is thicken enough.
4. Stir in the remaining oil, salt, and black pepper and remove the frying pan from heat and let it cool.
5. For crust: in a microwave-safe bowl, add the zucchini and microwave on High for about 5 minutes.
6. Place the zucchini into a colander lined with cheesecloth and set aside to cool.
7. Preheat the oven to 450 degrees F.
8. After the cooling, squeeze zucchini completely and transfer into a bowl.
9. In the bowl of zucchini, add the almond meal, grated mozzarella, Parmesan, egg, oregano, garlic powder, and salt and mix until well combined.
10. Divide the crust mixture into 2 balls and arrange onto a greased baking sheet.
11. With your fingers, press each crust ball into 2 circles. (Do not make edges too thin).
12. Arrange each crust onto a pizza stone and bake for about 12-13 minutes.
13. Remove crust from oven.
14. Spread the sauce evenly over each crust and top with the basil leaves and mozzarella chunks.
15. Bake for about 3-5 minutes.
16. Cut each pizza into 2 portions and serve hot.

## Nutrition Values (Per Serving)

- Calories: 263
- Net Carbs: 7.3g
- Carbohydrate: 11g
- Fiber: 3.7g
- Protein: 17.6g
- Fat: 17.1g
- Sugar: 5.4g
- Sodium: 370mg

---

# Spinach Pie

**(Yields:** 6 servings / **Prep Time:** 15 minutes / **Cooking Time:** 38 minutes)

## Ingredients

- 2 tablespoons unsalted butter, divided
- 2 tablespoons yellow onion, chopped
- 1 (16-ounces) package frozen chopped spinach, thawed and squeezed
- 1½ cups heavy cream

- 3 organic eggs
- ½ teaspoon ground nutmeg
- Salt and ground black pepper, as required
- ½ cup Swiss cheese, shredded

## Instructions

1. Preheat the oven to 375 degrees F and grease a 9-inch pie dish.
2. Melt 1 tablespoon of butter in a large skillet over medium-high heat and sauté the onion for about 4-5 minutes.
3. Add the spinach and cook for about 2-3 minutes or until all the liquid is absorbed.
4. Remove the skillet from heat and set aside.
5. Add the cream, eggs, nutmeg, salt, and black pepper in a bowl and beat until well combined.
6. Transfer the spinach mixture in the bottom of prepared pie dish.
7. Place the egg mixture evenly over spinach mixture and sprinkle with Swiss cheese.
8. Top with the remaining butter in the shape of dots at many places.
9. Bake for about 25-30 minutes or until the top becomes golden brown.
10. Remove the pie dish from oven and serve hot.

## Nutrition Values (Per Serving)

- Calories: 223
- Net Carbs: 2.8g
- Carbohydrate: 4.6g
- Fiber: 1.8g
- Protein: 8.1g
- Fat: 20g
- Sugar: 0.8g
- Sodium: 150mg

**(Tip:** Don't forget to thaw the frozen spinach before cooking.)

---

# Veggie Loaf

**(Yields:** 8 servings / **Prep Time:** 20 minutes / **Cooking Time:** 1 hour 10 minutes)

## Ingredients

- 1 tablespoon olive oil
- 2 yellow onions, chopped
- 2 garlic cloves, minced
- 1 teaspoon dried rosemary, crushed
- 1 cup walnuts, chopped
- 2 large carrots, peeled and chopped
- 1 large celery stalk, chopped
- 1 large green bell pepper, seeded and chopped
- 1 cup fresh button mushrooms, chopped
- 5 large organic eggs
- 1¼ cups almond flour
- Sea salt and ground black pepper, as required

## Instructions

1. Preheat the oven to 350 degrees F and line 2 loaf pans with lightly greased parchment papers.
2. Heat the oil in a large skillet over medium heat and sauté the onion for about 4-5 minutes.
3. Add the garlic, and rosemary and sauté for about 1 minute.
4. Add the walnuts, and vegetables and cook for about 3-4 minutes.
5. Remove the skillet from heat and transfer the mixture into a large bowl.
6. Set aside to cool slightly.
7. In another bowl, add the eggs, flour, sea salt, and black pepper and beat until well combined.
8. Add egg mixture into the bowl of vegetable mixture and mix until well combined.
9. Divide the mixture evenly into prepared loaf pans.
10. Bake for about 50-60 minutes or until the top becomes golden brown.
11. Remove from oven and cut the loaf into 8 equal-sized slices and serve.

## Nutrition Values (Per Serving)

- Calories: 208
- Net Carbs: 5.9g
- Carbohydrate: 8.9g
- Fiber: 3g
- Protein: 9.6g
- Fat: 16.4g
- Sugar: 3.6g
- Sodium: 80mg

---

# Curried Veggies Bake

**(Yields:** 6 servings / **Prep Time:** 20 minutes / **Cooking Time:** 20 minutes)

## Ingredients

- 1 medium zucchini, chopped
- 1 medium yellow squash, chopped
- 1 green bell pepper, seeded and cubed
- 1 red bell pepper, seeded and cubed
- 1 yellow onion, thinly sliced
- 2 tablespoons butter, melted
- 2 teaspoons red curry powder
- Salt and ground black pepper, as required
- ¼ cup homemade vegetable broth
- ¼ cup fresh cilantro leaves, finely chopped
- ½ cup Parmesan cheese, shredded

## Instructions

1. Preheat the oven to 375 degrees F and lightly, grease a large baking dish.
2. Add all the ingredients in a large bowl except cilantro, and Parmesan and mix until well combined.

3. Transfer the vegetable mixture into prepared baking dish.
4. Bake for about 15-20 minutes or until desired doneness of the vegetables.
5. Remove the vegetables from oven and immediately, sprinkle with the parmesan cheese.
6. Garnish with fresh cilantro and serve immediately.

## Nutrition Values (Per Serving)

- Calories: 96
- Net Carbs: 5.5g
- Carbohydrate: 7.4g
- Fiber: 1.9g
- Protein: 4.3g
- Fat: 6.1g
- Sugar: 4g
- Sodium: 181mg

---

# Mixed Veggies Stew

**(Yields:** 8 servings / **Prep Time:** 20 minutes / **Cooking Time:** 2¼ hours)

## Ingredients

- 2 tablespoons coconut oil
- 1 medium yellow onions, chopped
- 2 cups celery, chopped
- ½ teaspoon garlic, minced
- 3 cups fresh kale, tough ends removed and chopped
- ½ cup fresh mushroom, sliced
- 1 (15-ounces) can fire-roasted diced tomatoes
- 1 teaspoon dried rosemary
- 1 teaspoon dried sage
- 1 teaspoon dried oregano
- Salt and ground black pepper, as required
- 2 cups homemade vegetable broth
- 4 cups water

## Instructions

1. Melt the coconut oil in a large pan over medium heat and sauté the onion, celery, and garlic for about 5 minutes.
2. Add the remaining ingredients and stir to combine.
3. Increase the heat to high and bring to a boil.
4. Cook for about 10 minutes.
5. Now, lower the heat to medium and cook, covered for about 15 minutes.
6. Uncover the pan and cook for about 15 more minutes, stirring occasionally.
7. Now, lower the heat to low and simmer, covered for about 1½ hours.
8. Serve hot.

## Nutrition Values (Per Serving)

- Calories: 77
- Net Carbs: 6g
- Carbohydrate: 8.4g
- Fiber: 2.4g

- Protein: 3g
- Fat: 3.9g
- Sugar: 3g
- Sodium: 414mg

## Tofu & Veggies Stew

**(Yields:** 6 servings / **Prep Time:** 15 minutes / **Total Cooking Time:** 30 minutes)

## Ingredients

- 2 tablespoons garlic, peeled
- 1 jalapeño pepper, seeded and chopped
- 1 (16-ounces) jar roasted red peppers, rinsed, drained and chopped
- 2 cups vegetable broth
- 2 cups water
- 1 medium green bell pepper, seeded and thinly sliced
- 1 medium red bell pepper, seeded and thinly sliced
- 1 (16-ounces) package extra-firm tofu, drained and cubed
- 1 (10-ounces) package frozen baby spinach, thawed

## Instructions

1. Place the garlic, jalapeño pepper and roasted red peppers in a food processor and pulse until smooth.
2. In a large pan, add the peppers puree, broth, and water over medium-high heat and bring to a boil.
3. Add the bell peppers, and tofu and stir to combine.
4. Reduce the heat to medium and cook for about 5 minutes.
5. Stir in the spinach and cook for about 5 minutes.
6. Serve hot.

## Nutrition Values (Per Serving)

- Calories: 125
- Net Carbs: 7.5g
- Carbohydrate: 11g
- Fiber: 3.5g
- Protein: 11.7g
- Fat: 5.3g
- Sugar: 5g
- Sodium: 482mg

## Mixed Veggie Combo

**(Yields:** 6 servings / **Prep Time:** 15 minutes / **Cooking Time:** 12 minutes)

## Ingredients

- 3 tablespoons unsalted butter
- 1 pound frozen okra, thawed, trimmed and sliced
- 1 green bell pepper, seeded and chopped
- 2 celery stalks, chopped

- 1 small yellow onion, chopped
- 2 cups tomatoes, finely chopped
- Salt and ground black pepper, as required

## Instructions

1. In a large non-stick skillet, melt the butter over medium heat and sauté the okra, bell pepper, celery and onion for about 5-7 minutes.
2. Stir in the tomatoes, salt, and black pepper and cook for about 3-5 minutes.
3. Serve hot.

## Nutrition Values (Per Serving)

- Calories: 104
- Net Carbs: 6.2g
- Carbohydrate: 10g
- Fiber: 3.8g
- Protein: 2.4g
- Fat: 6.1g
- Sugar: 4.3g
- Sodium: 82mg

# Spinach in Cheese Sauce

**(Yields:** 4 servings / **Prep Time:** 10 minutes / **Cooking Time:** 15 minutes)

## Ingredients

- 2 tablespoons unsalted butter
- 1 medium yellow onion, chopped
- 1 cup cream cheese, softened
- 2 (10-ounces) packages frozen spinach, thawed and squeezed dry
- 2-3 tablespoons water
- Salt and ground black pepper, as required
- 2 teaspoons fresh lemon juice

## Instructions

1. Melt the butter in a skillet over medium heat and sauté the onion for about 6-8 minutes.
2. Add the cream cheese and cook for about 2 minutes or until melted completely.
3. Stir in the spinach, and water and cook for about 4-5 minutes.
4. Stir in salt, black pepper, and lemon juice and remove from the heat.
5. Serve immediately.

## Nutrition Values (Per Serving)

- Calories: 298
- Net Carbs: 5.6g
- Carbohydrate: 9.3g
- Fiber: 3.7g
- Protein: 8.8g
- Fat: 26.6g
- Sugar: 1.9g
- Sodium: 365mg

# Cheesy Cauliflower

**(Yields:** 4 servings / **Prep Time:** 10 minutes / **Cooking Time:** 30 minutes)

## Ingredients

- 1 head cauliflower
- 1 tablespoon prepared mustard
- 1 teaspoon mayonnaise
- ¼ cup butter, cut into small pieces
- ½ cup Parmesan cheese, grated

## Instructions

1. Preheat the oven to 375 degrees F.
2. Place the mustard and mayonnaise in a bowl and mix until well combined.
3. Coat the cauliflower head evenly with mustard mixture.
4. Arrange the cauliflower head into a baking dish and top with butter in the shape of dots, followed by Parmesan cheese.
5. Bake for about 30 minutes.
6. Remove from oven and cut the cauliflower head into desired size pieces and serve hot.

## Nutrition Values (Per Serving)

- Calories: 162
- Net Carbs: 2.2g
- Carbohydrate: 4g
- Fiber: 1.8g
- Protein: 5.6g
- Fat: 14.6g
- Sugar: 1.7g
- Sodium: 24mg

---

# Creamy Brussels Sprout

**(Yields:** 5 servings / **Prep Time:** 15 minutes / **Cooking Time:** 17 minutes)

## Ingredients

- 1½ pounds fresh Brussels sprouts, trimmed and halved
- 3 garlic cloves, minced
- 2 tablespoons butter, melted
- 2 tablespoons Dijon mustard
- ½ cup heavy whipping cream
- Salt and ground white pepper, as required

## Instructions

1. Preheat the oven to 450 degrees F.
2. In a large roasting pan, add the Brussels sprouts, garlic, and butter and toss to coat well.

3. Roast for about 10-15 minutes, tossing occasionally.
4. Meanwhile, add the remaining ingredients in a small pan over medium-low heat and bring to a gentle boil.
5. Cook for about 1-2 minutes, stirring continuously.
6. Serve Brussels sprouts with the topping of creamy sauce.

## Nutrition Values (Per Serving)

- Calories: 188
- Net Carbs: 7.8g
- Carbohydrate: 12.9g
- Fiber: 5.1g
- Protein: 4.8g
- Fat: 13.1g
- Sugar: 3g
- Sodium: 250mg

---

## Cauliflower & Cottage Cheese Curry

(**Yields:** 4 servings / **Prep Time:** 15 minutes / **Cooking Time:** 35 minutes)

## Ingredients

- 3 tablespoons butter
- 7 ounces cottage cheese, cut into 2-inch cubes
- ½ head cauliflower, cut into small florets
- ½ cup water
- 1 cup fresh cream
- ½ cup plain Greek yogurt
- 1-2 tablespoons curry paste
- 2 tablespoons fresh cilantro

## Instructions

1. In a large frying pan, melt half the butter over medium heat and stir fry the cottage cheese cubes for about 4-5 minutes or until golden from all sides.
2. With a slotted spoon, transfer the cheese cubes onto a plate and set aside.
3. In the same pan, melt the remaining butter and cook the cauliflower for about 2-3 minutes, stirring frequently.
4. Stir in the water and cook, covered for about 4-5 minutes until all the liquid is absorbed.
5. Meanwhile, place the cream, yogurt and curry paste in a bowl and beat until smooth.
6. Stir the yogurt mixture into the frying pan and simmer for about 15-20 minutes, stirring occasionally.
7. Stir in the fried cheese cubes and cook for about 2 minutes or until heated through.
8. Garnish with fresh cilantro and serve hot.

## Nutrition Values (Per Serving)

- Calories: 215
- Net Carbs: 7.2g
- Carbohydrate: 8.1g
- Fiber: 0.9g

- Protein: 10g
- Fat: 15.5g
- Sugar: 4.3g
- Sodium: 315mg

---

# Eggplant Curry

**(Yields:** 3 servings / **Prep Time:** 15 minutes / **Cooking Time:** 30 minutes)

## Ingredients

- 1 tablespoon coconut oil
- ½ of small yellow onion, finely chopped
- 2 small garlic cloves, minced
- ½ teaspoon fresh ginger root, minced
- 1 small Serrano pepper, seeded and minced
- 1 teaspoon curry powder
- ¼ teaspoon cayenne pepper
- 1 medium plum tomato, finely chopped
- 1 large eggplant, cubed
- Salt, as required
- ¾ cup unsweetened coconut milk
- 1 tablespoon fresh cilantro, chopped

## Instructions

1. Melt the coconut oil in a large skillet over medium heat and sauté the onion for about 5-6 minutes.
2. Add the garlic, ginger, Serrano pepper, and spices and sauté for about 1 minute.
3. Add the tomato and cook for about 3 minutes, crushing with the back of spoon.
4. Add the eggplant, and salt and cook for about 1 minute, stirring occasionally.
5. Stir in the coconut milk and bring to a gentle boil.
6. Lower the heat to medium-low and simmer, covered for about 20 minutes or until done completely.
7. Garnish with fresh cilantro and serve.

## Nutrition Values (Per Serving)

- Calories: 109
- Net Carbs: 6.2g
- Carbohydrate: 13g
- Fiber: 6.8g
- Protein: 2.3g
- Fat: 6g
- Sugar: 5g
- Sodium: 58mg

# Curried Broccoli

**(Yields:** 4 servings / **Prep Time:** 15 minutes / **Cooking Time:** 15 minutes)

## Ingredients

- ¼ cup unsweetened coconut flakes
- 1 tablespoon coconut oil
- ½ of small yellow onion, thinly sliced
- 1 tablespoon fresh ginger, minced
- 2 teaspoons curry powder
- 1 teaspoon cumin seeds
- Salt, as required
- 2 tablespoons water
- 1 pound fresh broccoli florets

## Instructions

1. Heat a large nonstick skillet over medium heat and cook the coconut flakes for about 3-4 minutes, stirring continuously.
2. Transfer the toasted coconut flakes into a bowl and set aside.
3. In the same skillet, melt the coconut oil over medium heat and sauté the onion for about 3-4 minutes.
4. Add the ginger, and spices and sauté for about 1-2 minutes.
5. Add the water, and broccoli and stir to combine.
6. Increase the heat to medium-high and cook, covered for about 3-4 minutes.
7. Top with the toasted coconut flakes and serve hot.

## Nutrition Values (Per Serving)

- Calories: 99
- Net Carbs: 6.8g
- Carbohydrate: 11g
- Fiber: 4.2g
- Protein: 3.9g
- Fat: 5.6g
- Sugar: 2.4g
- Sodium: 79mg

---

# Stuffed Zucchini

**(Yields:** 8 servings / **Prep Time:** 15 minutes / **Cooking Time:** 18 minutes)

## Ingredients

- 4 medium zucchinis, halved lengthwise
- 1 cup red bell pepper, seeded and minced
- ½ cup Kalamata olives, pitted and minced
- ½ cup fresh tomatoes, minced
- 1 teaspoon garlic, minced
- 1 tablespoon dried oregano, crushed
- Salt and ground black pepper, as required
- ½ cup feta cheese, crumbled
- ¼ cup fresh parsley, finely chopped

### Instructions

1. Preheat the oven to 350 degrees F and grease a large baking sheet.
2. With a melon baller, scoop out the flesh of each zucchini half. Discard the flesh.
3. In a bowl, mix together the bell pepper, olives, tomatoes, garlic, oregano, salt and black pepper.
4. Stuff each zucchini half evenly with the veggie mixture.
5. Arrange zucchini halves onto the prepared baking sheet and bake for about 15 minutes.
6. Now, set the oven to broiler on high.
7. Top each zucchini half with feta cheese and broil for about 3 minutes.
8. Garnish with fresh parsley and serve hot.

### Nutrition Values (Per Serving)

- Calories: 60
- Net Carbs: 4.4g
- Carbohydrate: 6.4g
- Fiber: 2g
- Protein: 3g
- Fat: 3.2g
- Sugar: 3.2g
- Sodium: 190mg

===

## Stuffed Bell Peppers

**(Yields:** 4 servings / **Prep Time:** 15 minutes / **Cooking Time:** 50 minutes)

### Ingredients

- 4 large organic eggs
- ½ cup plus 2 tablespoons Parmesan cheese, grated and divided
- ½ cup mozzarella cheese, shredded
- ½ cup ricotta cheese
- 1 teaspoon garlic powder
- ¼ teaspoon dried parsley
- 2 medium bell peppers, cut in half and seeded
- ¼ cup fresh baby spinach leaves

### Instructions

1. Preheat the oven to 375 degrees F and lightly, grease a baking dish.
2. In a small food processor, place the eggs, ½ cup of Parmesan, mozzarella, ricotta cheese, garlic powder, and parsley and pulse until well combined.
3. Arrange the bell pepper halves into prepared baking dish, cut side up.
4. Place the cheese mixture into each pepper half and top each with few spinach leaves.
5. With a fork, push the spinach leaves into cheese mixture.
6. With a piece of foil, cover the baking dish and bake for about 35-45 minutes.
7. Now, set the oven to broiler on high.

8. Top each bell pepper half with the remaining Parmesan cheese and broil for about 3-5 minutes.
9. Remove from the oven and serve hot.

## Nutrition Values (Per Serving)
- Calories: 191
- Net Carbs: 6g
- Carbohydrate: 7g
- Fiber: 1g
- Protein: 16.6g
- Fat: 11.2g
- Sugar: 3.7g
- Sodium: 241mg

---

# Bell Pepper with Yellow Squash

**(Yields:** 4 servings / **Prep Time:** 10 minutes / **Cooking Time:** 10 minutes)

## Ingredients
- 1 tablespoon butter
- ½ cup yellow onion, sliced
- ½ cup red bell pepper, seeded and julienned
- ½ cup green bell pepper, seeded and julienned
- 3 cups yellow squash, sliced
- 1½ teaspoons garlic, minced
- ¼ cup water
- Salt and ground black pepper, as required

## Instructions
1. Melt the butter in a large skillet over medium-high heat and sauté the onion, bell peppers and squash for about 4-5 minutes.
2. Add the garlic and sauté for about 1 minute.
3. Add the remaining ingredients and stir to combine.
4. Reduce the heat to medium and cook for about 3-4 minutes, stirring occasionally.
5. Serve hot.

## Nutrition Values (Per Serving)
- Calories: 60
- Net Carbs: 6g
- Carbohydrate: 7.7g
- Fiber: 1.7g
- Protein: 1.8g
- Fat: 3.1g
- Sugar: 3.6g
- Sodium: 70mg

# Braised Cabbage

**(Yields:** 3 servings / **Prep Time:** 10 minutes / **Cooking Time:** 25 minutes)

## Ingredients

- 1½ teaspoons butter
- 2½ cups green cabbage, chopped
- 1 garlic clove, chopped
- 1 yellow onion, thinly sliced
- 1 cup homemade vegetable broth
- Salt, as required

## Instructions

1. Melt the butter in a large nonstick skillet over high heat and sauté the cabbage, garlic and onion for about 5 minutes.
2. Gradually, stir in the broth and immediately, reduce the heat to low.
3. Stir in salt and cook, covered for about 20 minutes.
4. Serve hot.

## Nutrition Values (Per Serving)

- Calories: 45
- Net Carbs: 3.9g
- Carbohydrate: 5.6g
- Fiber: 1.7g
- Protein: 2.1g
- Fat: 1.8g
- Sugar: 2.8g
- Sodium: 249mg

---

# Salad Wraps

**(Yields:** 4 servings / **Prep Time:** 15 minutes / **Cooking Time:** 15 minutes)

## Ingredients

- 1 tablespoon olive oil
- 1 teaspoon cumin seeds
- 1 small yellow onion, thinly sliced
- 4 cups zucchini, grated
- ½ teaspoon red pepper flakes, crushed
- Salt and ground black pepper, as required
- 8 large lettuce leaves, rinsed and pat dried
- ¼ cup Parmesan cheese, shredded
- 2 tablespoons fresh chives, finely minced

## Instructions

1. In a medium skillet, heat the oil over medium-high heat and sauté the cumin seeds for about 1 minute.
2. Add the onion and sauté for about 4-5 minutes.

3. Add the zucchini and cook for about 5-7 minutes or until done completely, stirring occasionally.
4. Stir in the red pepper flakes, salt, and black pepper and remove from the heat.
5. Arrange the lettuce leaves onto a smooth surface.
6. Divide the zucchini mixture evenly onto each lettuce leaf.
7. Top with the Parmesan and fresh chives and serve immediately.

## Nutrition Values (Per Serving)

- Calories: 80
- Net Carbs: 3g
- Carbohydrate: 6.7g
- Fiber: 3.7g
- Protein: 3.7g
- Fat: 5.3g
- Sugar: 2.9g
- Sodium: 137mg

# Creamy Zucchini Noodles

**(Yields:** 4 servings / **Prep Time:** 15 minutes / **Cooking Time:** 10 minutes)

## Ingredients

- 1¼ cups heavy whipping cream
- ¼ cup mayonnaise
- Salt and ground black pepper, as required
- 30 ounces zucchini, spiralized with blade C
- 4 organic egg yolks
- 3 ounces Parmesan cheese, grated
- 2 tablespoons fresh parsley, chopped
- 2 tablespoons butter, melted

## Instructions

1. In a pan, add the heavy cream and bring to a boil.
2. Lower the heat to low and cook until reduced in half.
3. Add the mayonnaise, salt, and black pepper and cook until mixture is warm enough.
4. Add the zucchini noodles and gently, stir to combine.
5. Top the zucchini noodle mixture with egg yolks and immediately, remove from the heat.
6. Place the zucchini noodles mixture evenly onto 4 serving plates and immediately, sprinkle with the parmesan and fresh parsley.
7. Drizzle with the melted butter and serve.

## Nutrition Values (Per Serving)

- Calories: 342
- Net Carbs: 5.6g
- Carbohydrate: 7.5g
- Fiber: 1.9g
- Protein: 10.4g
- Fat: 31.3g
- Sugar: 3.1g
- Sodium: 329mg

# Buttered Yellow Squash Noodles

**(Yields:** 4 servings / **Prep Time:** 15 minutes / **Cooking Time:** 12 minutes)

## Ingredients

- 2 tablespoons butter
- 1 yellow onion, thinly sliced
- 4 small yellow squashes, spiralized with blade C
- ¼ cup sugar-free barbecue sauce

## Instructions

1. Melt the butter in a large skillet over medium heat and sauté the onion for about 4-5 minutes.
2. Add the squash noodles and cook for about 2 minutes.
3. Stir in barbeque sauce and cook for about 3-5 minutes or until desired doneness.
4. Serve hot.

## Nutrition Values (Per Serving)

- Calories: 98
- Net Carbs: 7.2g
- Carbohydrate: 10g
- Fiber: 2.8g
- Protein: 2.8g
- Fat: 6.1g
- Sugar: 5g
- Sodium: 72mg

---

# Grilled Zucchini

**(Yields:** 2 servings / **Prep Time:** 10 minutes / **Cooking Time:** 8 minutes)

## Ingredients

- 1 large zucchini, cut into ¼-inch slices
- ¼ cup Italian-style salad dressing

## Instructions

1. Preheat the grill to medium-low heat. Grease the grill grate.
2. In a bowl, add the zucchini and salad dressing and toss to coat.
3. Grill the zucchini slices for about 3-4 minutes per side.
4. Serve hot.

## Nutrition Values (Per Serving)

- Calories: 111
- Net Carbs: 6.3g
- Carbohydrate: 8g
- Fiber: 1.7g
- Protein: 2.1g
- Fat: 8.6g
- Sugar: 5g
- Sodium: 503mg

# Garlicky Broccoli

**(Yields:** 3 servings / **Prep Time:** 10 minutes / **Total Cooking Time:** 10 minutes)

## Ingredients

- 2 tablespoons butter
- 2 garlic cloves, minced
- 2½ cups broccoli florets
- 2-3 tablespoons low-sodium soy sauce
- 1/8 teaspoon red pepper flakes

## Instructions

1. Melt the butter in a large skillet over medium heat and sauté the garlic for about 1 minute.
2. Add the broccoli and stir fry for about 2-3 minutes.
3. Stir in the soy sauce and stir fry for about 4-5 minutes.
4. Serve hot.

## Nutrition Values (Per Serving)

- Calories: 100
- Net Carbs: 4.4g
- Carbohydrate: 6.4g
- Fiber: 2g
- Protein: 3g
- Fat: 8g
- Sugar: 2g
- Sodium: 667mg

---

# Lemony Brussels Sprout

**(Yields:** 2 servings / **Prep Time:** 10 minutes / **Cooking Time:** 15 minutes)

## Ingredients

- ½ pound Brussels sprouts, halved
- 1 tablespoon olive oil
- 2 garlic cloves, minced
- ½ teaspoon red pepper flakes, crushed
- Salt and ground black pepper, as required
- 1 tablespoon fresh lemon juice

## Instructions

1. Arrange a steamer basket over a large pan of boiling filtered water.
2. Place the Brussels sprout in steamer basket and steam, covered for about 6-8 minutes.
3. Drain the Brussels sprout well.
4. Heat the olive oil in a large skillet over medium heat and sauté the garlic and red pepper flakes for about 1 minute.
5. Add the Brussels sprouts, salt, and black pepper and sauté for 4 to 5 minutes.

6. Stir in lemon juice and sauté for 1 more minute.
7. Serve hot.

## Nutrition Values (Per Serving)

- Calories: 115
- Net Carbs: 6.8g
- Carbohydrate: 11.2g
- Fiber: 4.4g
- Protein: 4.1g
- Fat: 7.5g
- Sugar: 2.5g
- Sodium: 102mg

## Buttered Asparagus

**(Yields:** 5 servings / **Prep Time:** 10 minutes / **Cooking Time:** 6 minutes)

## Ingredients

- 2 tablespoons butter
- 1 teaspoon cumin seed
- 2 pounds fresh asparagus, trimmed and cut into 2-inch pieces diagonally
- 1 tablespoon fresh ginger, minced
- 2 teaspoons fresh lemon juice
- Salt and ground black pepper, as required

## Instructions

1. Heat the butter in a skillet over medium heat and sauté the cumin seeds for about 1 minute.
2. Add the remaining ingredients and stir fry for about 4-5 minutes.
3. Serve warm.

## Nutrition Values (Per Serving)

- Calories: 83
- Net Carbs: 7.2g
- Carbohydrate: 10g
- Fiber: 2.8g
- Protein: 4.2g
- Fat: 5g
- Sugar: 3.5g
- Sodium: 160mg

## Spiced mushroom

**(Yields:** 2 servings / **Prep Time:** 15 minutes / **Cooking Time:** 16 minutes)

## Ingredients

- 2 tablespoons butter
- ½ teaspoon cumin seeds, lightly crushed
- 1 yellow onion, thinly sliced
- ½ pound white button mushrooms, chopped

- 1 green chili, chopped
- 1 teaspoon ground coriander
- ½ teaspoon garam masala powder
- ½ teaspoon red chili powder
- 1/8 teaspoon ground turmeric
- Salt, as required
- 2 tablespoons fresh cilantro leaves, chopped

## Instructions

1. Melt the butter in a skillet over medium heat and sauté the cumin seeds for about 1 minute.
2. Add the onion and sauté for about 4-5 minutes.
3. Add the mushrooms and sauté for about 5-7 minutes.
4. Add the green chili, spices, and salt and sauté for about 1-2 minutes.
5. Stir in the cilantro and sauté for about 1 more minute.
6. Serve hot.

## Nutrition Values (Per Serving)

- Calories: 154
- Net Carbs: 7g
- Carbohydrate: 9.8g
- Fiber: 2.8g
- Protein: 4.6g
- Fat: 12.2g
- Sugar: 4.5g
- Sodium: 177mg

---

# Cauliflower Mash

**(Yields:** 6 servings / **Prep Time:** 15 minutes / **Cooking Time:** 12 minutes)

## Ingredients

- 1 large head cauliflower, cut into florets
- 1/3 cup heavy whipping cream
- 1 cup Parmesan cheese, shredded and divided
- 1 tablespoon butter
- Freshly ground black pepper, as required
- 1 tablespoon fresh parsley, chopped

## Instructions

1. In a large pan of boiling water, add the cauliflower and cook, covered for about 10-12 minutes.
2. Drain the cauliflower well.
3. Place the cauliflower, cream, ½ cup of cheese, butter and black pepper in a large food processor and pulse until smooth.
4. Transfer the cauliflower mash into a bowl.
5. Top with the remaining cheese, and parsley and serve

### Nutrition Values (Per Serving)

- Calories: 107
- Net Carbs: 2.1g
- Carbohydrate: 3g
- Fiber: 1.1g
- Protein: 6.1g
- Fat: 8.1g
- Sugar: 1.1g
- Sodium: 256mg

## Broccoli Mash

**(Yields:** 6 servings / **Prep Time:** 15 minutes / **Cooking Time:** 5 minutes)

### Ingredients

- 16 ounces broccoli florets
- 1 cup water
- 1 teaspoon fresh lemon juice
- 1 teaspoon butter, softened
- 1 teaspoon garlic, minced
- Salt and ground black pepper, as required

### Instructions

1. In a medium pan, add the broccoli and water over medium heat and cook for about 5 minutes.
2. Drain the broccoli well and transfer into a large bowl.
3. In the bowl of broccoli, add the lemon juice, butter, and garlic and with an immersion blender blend until smooth.
4. Season with salt and black pepper and serve.

### Nutrition Values (Per Serving)

- Calories: 32
- Net Carbs: 3.1g
- Carbohydrate: 5.1g
- Fiber: 2g
- Protein: 2g
- Fat: 0.9g
- Sugar: 1.3g
- Sodium: 160mg

# CHAPTER 9 | DESSERTS & DRINKS

## Mocha Ice Cream

**(Yields:** 2 servings / **Prep Time:** 15 minutes)

### Ingredients

- 1 cup unsweetened coconut milk
- ¼ cup heavy cream
- 2 tablespoons Erythritol
- 15 drops liquid stevia
- 2 tablespoons cacao powder
- 1 tablespoon instant coffee
- ¼ teaspoon xanthan gum

### Instructions

1. In a container, add all the ingredients except xanthan gum and with an immersion blender, blend until well combined.
2. Slowly, add the xanthan gum and blend until a slightly thicker mixture is formed.
3. Transfer the mixture into ice cream maker and process according to the manufacturer's instructions.
4. Now, transfer the ice cream into an airtight container and freeze for at least 4-5 hours before serving.

### Nutrition Values (Per Serving)

- Calories: 339
- Net Carbs: 5.4g
- Carbohydrate: 10g
- Fiber: 4.6g
- Protein: 4.1g
- Fat: 35.2g
- Sugar: 4g
- Sodium: 33mg

**(Tip:** Strictly follow the ratio of ingredients.)

## Coffee Granita

**(Yields:** 8 servings / **Prep Time:** 10 minutes)

### Ingredients

- 4 cups hot brewed extra strong coffee
- 2 teaspoons ground cinnamon
- ½ cup Erythritol
- 1¼ cups heavy cream, divided

### Instructions

1. Place the coffee, cinnamon and Erythritol in a large bowl and stir until sweetener is completely dissolved.
2. Add ¼ cup of cream and beat until well combined.
3. Refrigerate for about 30 minutes.

4. Remove from refrigerator and transfer the mixture into a shallow baking dish.
5. Freeze for about 3 hours, scraping after every 30 minutes with the help of a fork.
6. With a foil paper, cover tightly and freeze before serving.
7. While serving, in a bowl, add the remaining cream and beat until soft peaks form.
8. Place the granita in serving glasses.
9. Add the whipped cream evenly over each glass and serve.

## Nutrition Values (Per Serving)

- Calories: 67
- Net Carbs: 0.7g
- Carbohydrate: 1g
- Fiber: 0.3g
- Protein: 0.5g
- Fat: 7g
- Sugar: 0g
- Sodium: 10mg

---

# Strawberry Sundae

**(Yields:** 1 serving / **Prep Time:** 10 minutes)

## Ingredients

- ¼ cup ricotta cheese
- 1 teaspoon organic vanilla extract
- 1 teaspoon fresh lemon juice
- 2 drops liquid stevia
- ¼ cup fresh strawberries, hulled and sliced
- 1 teaspoon almonds, chopped

## Instructions:

1. In a bowl, add all the ingredients except strawberries and beat until smooth.
2. In a serving glass, place half of cheese mixture. Place strawberries over cheese mixture.
3. Top with remaining cheese mixture and serve immediately.

## Nutrition Values (Per Serving)

- Calories: 122
- Net Carbs: 6g
- Carbohydrate: 7g
- Fiber: 1g
- Protein: 7.8g
- Fat: 6g
- Sugar: 2.7g
- Sodium: 79mg

# Chocolate Pudding

**(Yields:** 4 servings / **Prep Time:** 15 minutes / **Total Cooking Time:** 5 minutes)

## Ingredients

- 1/3 cup Erythritol
- ¼ teaspoon stevia powder
- ¼ cup cacao powder
- 2 cups unsweetened coconut milk
- ¼ cup heavy cream
- 1 teaspoon xanthan gum
- 2 tablespoons butter
- 1 teaspoon organic vanilla extract

## Instructions

1. Place the Erythritol, stevia powder, and cacao powder in a pan and mix well.
2. Slowly, add the coconut milk and heavy cream, stirring continuously until well combined.
3. Place the pan over medium heat and bring to a boil, stirring continuously.
4. Cook for about 1 minute, stirring continuously.
5. Remove the pan of cream mixture from heat and stir in the xanthan gum until well combined.
6. Add the butter and vanilla extract and mix until well combined.
7. Transfer the mixture into a large bowl.
8. With a plastic wrap, cover the surface of pudding and refrigerate to chill before serving.
9. Remove from the refrigerator and with an electric mixer, beat the pudding until smooth.
10. Serve immediately.

## Nutrition Values (Per Serving)

- Calories: 372
- Net Carbs: 5g
- Carbohydrate: 10g
- Fiber: 5g
- Protein: 4g
- Fat: 38.2g
- Sugar: 4.2g
- Sodium: 79mg

# Mascarpone Custard

**(Yields:** 4 servings / **Prep Time:** 15 minutes / **Cooking Time:** 8 minutes)

## Ingredients

- ¼ cup unsalted butter
- 4 ounces mascarpone cream cheese
- 4 large organic eggs (whites and yolks separated)
- 1 teaspoon espresso powder
- 1 tablespoon water
- ¼ teaspoon cream of tartar
- ¼ teaspoon monk fruit extract drops
- ½ teaspoon liquid stevia

## Instructions

1. Place the butter and cream cheese in a medium pan over medium-low heat and cook for about 2-3 minutes or until melted completely, stirring continuously.
2. Add the egg yolks, espresso powder, and water and stir to combine.
3. Adjust the heat to low and simmer for about 2-4 minutes or until desired thickness, stirring continuously.
4. Meanwhile, in a bowl, add cream of tartar and egg whites and beat until stiff peaks form.
5. Remove from the heat and immediately, stir in fruit extract drops and stevia.
6. Gently, fold in the egg white mixture.
7. Transfer into serving glasses and refrigerate to chill before serving.

## Nutrition Values (Per Serving)

- Calories: 223
- Net Carbs: 1.4g
- Carbohydrate: 1.4g
- Fiber: 0g
- Protein: 9.6g
- Fat: 20.2g
- Sugar: 0.5g
- Sodium: 176mg

---

# Vanilla Crème Brûlée

**(Yields:** 4 servings / **Prep Time:** 20 minutes / **Cooking Time:** 1 hour)

## Ingredients

- 2 cups heavy cream
- 1 vanilla bean, halved and scraped out seeds
- 4 organic egg yolks
- 1/3 teaspoon stevia powder
- 1 teaspoon organic vanilla extract
- Pinch of salt
- 4 tablespoons granulated Erythritol

## Instructions

1. Preheat the oven to 350 degrees F.
2. Place the heavy cream in a pan over medium heat and cook until heated.
3. Stir in the vanilla bean seeds and bring to a gentle boil.
4. Adjust the heat to very-low and cook, covered for about 20 minutes.
5. Meanwhile, in a bowl, add the remaining ingredients except Erythritol and beat until thick and pale mixture forms.
6. Remove the heavy cream from heat and through a fine mesh strainer, strain into a heatproof bowl.
7. Slowly, add the cream in egg yolk mixture beating continuously until well combined.
8. Divide the mixture into 4 ramekins.

9. Arrange the ramekins into a large baking dish.
10. In the baking dish, add hot water about half way of the ramekins.
11. Bake for about 30-35 minutes.
12. Remove the baking dish from oven and let the ramekins cool slightly.
13. Refrigerate the ramekins for at least 4 hours.
14. Just before serving, sprinkle the ramekins evenly with Erythritol.
15. Holding a kitchen torch about 4-5-inch from the top, caramelize the Erythritol for about 2 minutes.
16. Set aside for 5 minutes before serving.

## **Nutrition Values (Per Serving)**

- Calories: 264
- Net Carbs: 2.4g
- Carbohydrate: 2.4g
- Fiber: 0g
- Protein: 3.9g
- Fat: 26.7g
- Sugar: 0.3g
- Sodium: 31mg

# Lemon Soufflé

(**Yields:** 4 servings / **Prep Time:** 15 minutes / **Cooking Time:** 20 minutes)

## **Ingredients**

- 2 large organic eggs (whites and yolks separated)
- ¼ cup Erythritol, divided
- 1 cup ricotta cheese
- 1 tablespoon fresh lemon juice
- 2 teaspoons lemon zest, grated
- 1 teaspoon poppy seeds
- 1 teaspoon organic vanilla extract

## **Instructions**

1. Preheat the oven to 375 degrees F. Grease 4 ramekins.
2. In a clean glass bowl, add the egg whites and beat until foamy.
3. Add 2 tablespoons of Erythritol and beat until stiff peaks form.
4. In another bowl, add the ricotta cheese, egg yolks and remaining Erythritol and beat until well combined.
5. Now, place the lemon juice, and lemon zest and mix well.
6. Add the poppy seeds, and vanilla extract and mix until well combined.
7. Add the whipped egg whites into ricotta mixture and gently, stir to combine.
8. Place the mixture evenly into prepared ramekins.
9. Bake for about 20 minutes.
10. Remove from the oven and serve immediately.

### Nutrition Values (Per Serving)

- Calories: 130
- Net Carbs: g
- Carbohydrate: 4g
- Fiber: 0.2g
- Protein: 10.4g
- Fat: 7.7g
- Sugar: 0.2g
- Sodium: 112mg

---

## Chocolate Panna Cota

**(Yields:** 4 servings / **Prep Time:** 15 minutes / **Cooking Time:** 5 minutes)

### Ingredients

- 1½ cups unsweetened almond milk, divided
- 1 tablespoon unflavored powdered gelatin
- 1 cup unsweetened coconut milk
- 1/3 cup Swerve
- 3 tablespoons cacao powder
- 2 teaspoons instant coffee granules
- 6 drops liquid stevia

### Instructions

1. In a large bowl, add ½ cup of almond milk and sprinkle evenly with gelatin. Set aside until soaked.
2. In a pan, add the remaining almond milk, coconut milk, Swerve, cacao powder, coffee granules, and stevia and bring to a gentle boil, stirring continuously.
3. Remove from the heat.
4. In a blender, add the gelatin mixture, and hot milk mixture and pulse until smooth.
5. Transfer the mixture into serving glasses and set aside to cool completely.
6. With plastic wrap, cover each glass and refrigerate for about 3-4 hours before serving.

### Nutrition Values (Per Serving)

- Calories: 136
- Net Carbs: 4.3g
- Carbohydrate: 5.8g
- Fiber: 1.5g
- Protein: 4.4g
- Fat: 12.1g
- Sugar: 1g
- Sodium: 96mg

# Cream Cheese Flan

**(Yields:** 8 servings / **Prep Time:** 15 minutes / **Cooking Time:** 1 hour 5 minutes)

## Ingredients

- ¾ cup granulated Erythritol, divided
- 3 tablespoons water, divided
- 2 teaspoons organic vanilla extract, divided
- 5 large organic eggs
- 2 cups heavy whipping cream
- 8 ounces full-fat cream cheese, softened
- ¼ teaspoon sea salt

## Instructions

1. Preheat the oven to 350 degrees F. Grease an 8-inch cake pan.
2. For caramel: in a heavy-bottomed pan, add ½ cup of Erythritol, 2 tablespoons of water and 1 teaspoon of vanilla extract over medium-low heat and cook until sweetener is melted completely, stirring continuously.
3. Remove the pan from heat and place caramel in the bottom of prepared cake pan.
4. In a blender, add the remaining Erythritol, water, vanilla extract, heavy cream, cream cheese, eggs, and salt and pulse until smooth.
5. Place the cream cheese mixture evenly over caramel.
6. Arrange the cake pan into a large roasting pan.
7. In the roasting pan, add hot water about 1-inch up sides of the cake pan.
8. Place the roasting pan in oven and bake for about 1 hour or until center becomes set.
9. Remove the cake pan from oven and place the cake pan in water bath to cool completely.
10. Refrigerate for about 4-5 hours before serving.

## Nutrition Values (Per Serving)

- Calories: 250
- Net Carbs: 2g
- Carbohydrate: 2g
- Fiber: 0g
- Protein: 6.7g
- Fat: 24.1g
- Sugar: 0.5g
- Sodium: 198mg

# Cream Fudge

**(Yields:** 24 servings / **Prep Time:** 15 minutes / **Total Cooking Time:** 25 minutes)

## Ingredients

- 2 cups heavy whipping cream
- 1 teaspoon organic vanilla extract
- 3 ounces butter, softened
- 3 ounces 70% dark chocolate, finely chopped

## Instructions

1. In a heavy-bottomed pan, add the heavy cream, and vanilla and bring to a full rolling boil.
2. Adjust the heat to low and simmer for about 20 minutes, stirring occasionally.
3. Add the butter and stir until smooth.
4. Remove the pan from heat and stir in the chopped chocolate until melted completely.
5. Place the mixture into a 7x7-inch baking dish.
6. Refrigerate until set completely.
7. Cut into 24 equal-sized pieces and serve cold.

## Nutrition Values (Per Serving)

- Calories: 79
- Net Carbs: 2.3g
- Carbohydrate: 2.4g
- Fiber: 0.1g
- Protein: 0.5g
- Fat: 7.6g
- Sugar: 1.9g
- Sodium: 27mg

---

# Cream Tartlets

**(Yields:** 6 servings / **Prep Time:** 20 minutes / **Cooking Time:** 10 minutes)

## Ingredients

**For Crust:**
- 2¼ cups almond flour
- ¼ cup powdered Swerve
- 5 tablespoons butter, melted
- ¼ teaspoon sea salt

**For Garnishing:**
- ½ cup fresh strawberries, hulled

**For Mascarpone Cream:**
- 6 ounces mascarpone cheese, softened
- 2 tablespoons powdered Erythritol
- 1/3 cup heavy cream
- ¼ teaspoon fresh lemon zest, grated
- 1 teaspoon organic vanilla extract

## Instructions

1. Preheat the oven to 350 degrees F. Grease 6 (4-inch) tart pans.
2. For crust: in a bowl, add all the ingredients and mix until well combined.
3. Place the dough evenly into prepared tart pans and with your hands, press the mixture in the bottom and up sides.
4. With a fork, prick the bottom of all crusts.
5. Bake for about 8-10 minutes.
6. Remove from the oven and place onto a wire rack to cool completely.

7. For the mascarpone cream: in a bowl, add mascarpone cheese, and Erythritol and with a mixer, beat on low speed for about 2 minutes.
8. Slowly, add the heavy cream, beating continuously on low speed until well combined.
9. Now, beat on high speed for about 30-60 seconds or until thick.
10. Add the lemon zest, and vanilla extract and beat until well combined.
11. Transfer the mascarpone cream into a piping bag, fitted with a large star shaped tip and fill the tartlets.
12. Garnish with fresh strawberries and serve.

## Nutrition Values (Per Serving)

- Calories: 414
- Net Carbs: 6g
- Carbohydrate: 10.8g
- Fiber: 4.8g
- Protein: 12.5g
- Fat: 35.7g
- Sugar: 0.6g
- Sodium: 188mg

## Blackberry Cobbler

**(Yields:** 8 servings / **Prep Time:** 15 minutes / **Cooking Time:** 22 minutes)

## Ingredients

### For Filling:
- 3 cups fresh blueberries
- 2 tablespoons Swerve
- ¼ teaspoon xanthan gum
- 1 teaspoon fresh lemon juice

### For Topping:
- 2/3 cup almond flour
- 2 tablespoons Swerve
- 2 tablespoons butter, melted
- ½ teaspoon fresh lemon zest, grated finely

## Instructions

1. Preheat the oven to 375 degrees F.
2. For filling: place all the ingredients in a bowl and mix well.
3. For the topping: add all the ingredients in another bowl and mix until a crumbly mixture forms.
4. Place the filling mixture into a 9x9-inch pie dish.
5. Place the topping mixture over the filling mixture.
6. Bake for about 22 minutes or until the top becomes golden brown.
7. Remove the pie dish from oven and set aside to cool slightly.
8. Cut into 8 equal-sized portions and serve warm.

## Nutrition Values (Per Serving)

- Calories: 108
- Net Carbs: 4.3g
- Carbohydrate: 8.3g
- Fiber: 4g

- Protein: 2.8g
- Fat: 7.6g
- Sugar: 2.7g
- Sodium: 27mg

---

# No-Bake Cheesecake

**(Yields:** 8 servings / **Prep Time:** 20 minutes)

## Ingredients

**For Crust:**
- ¾ cup unsweetened coconut, shredded
- ¾ cup raw sunflower seeds
- ¼ cup Erythritol
- ¼ teaspoon salt
- 3 tablespoons unsalted butter, melted

**For Filling:**
- 2 cups fresh strawberries, hulled and sliced
- 1½ teaspoons fresh lemon juice
- 1 teaspoon liquid stevia
- ¼ teaspoon salt
- 8 ounces cream cheese, softened
- ½ teaspoon organic vanilla extract
- 1 cup heavy cream

## Instructions

1. For crust: place the coconut, sunflower seeds, Erythritol and salt in a food processor and pulse until a fine crumb like mixture is formed.
2. While motor is running, add the butter and pulse until well combined.
3. Transfer the mixture into a 9-inch pie dish and with your hands, press the mixture in the bottom and up sides of pie dish.
4. With a paper towel, wipe out the blender.
5. Now in the clean blender, add the strawberries, lemon juice, stevia, and salt and pulse until a puree forms.
6. Transfer the strawberry puree into a bowl.
7. Place the cream cheese in another bowl and beat until smooth.
8. Add the vanilla and heavy cream and beat until fluffy.
9. Add the strawberry puree mixture and mix until well combined.
10. Place strawberry mixture over the crust mixture and freeze for at least 4-8 hours.
11. Remove from the freezer and set aside for about 5 minutes.
12. Cut into 8 equal-sized slices and serve.

## Nutrition Values (Per Serving)

- Calories: 254
- Net Carbs: 4.2g
- Carbohydrate: 6g
- Fiber: 1.8g
- Protein: 3.9g
- Fat: 24.6g
- Sugar: 2.5g
- Sodium: 196mg

# Cream Cake

**(Yields:** 12 servings / **Prep Time:** 15 minutes / **Cooking Time:** 50 minutes)

## Ingredients

- 2 cups almond flour
- 2 teaspoons organic baking powder
- ½ cup butter, chopped
- 2 ounces cream cheese, softened
- 1 cup sour cream
- 1 cup Erythritol
- 1 teaspoon organic vanilla extract
- 4 large organic eggs

## Instructions

1. Preheat the oven to 350 degrees F. Generously, grease a 9-inch Bundt pan.
2. Place the almond flour and baking powder in a large bowl and mix well. Set aside.
3. In a microwave-safe bowl, add the butter and cream cheese and microwave for about 30 seconds.
4. Remove from the microwave and stir well.
5. In the bowl of butter mixture, add the sour cream, Erythritol, and vanilla extract and mix until well combined.
6. Add the butter mixture into the bowl of flour mixture and mix until well combined.
7. Now, add the eggs and mix until well combined.
8. Transfer the mixture evenly into the prepared pan.
9. Bake for about 48-50 minutes or until a toothpick inserted in the center comes out clean.
10. Remove the pan from oven and place onto a wire rack to cool completely.
11. Carefully, invert the cake onto a wire rack to cool completely.
12. Cut into 12 equal-sized slices and serve.

## Nutrition Values (Per Serving)

- Calories: 263
- Net Carbs: 3.5g
- Carbohydrate: 5.5g
- Fiber: 2g
- Protein: 7.2g
- Fat: 23.9g
- Sugar: 0.2g
- Sodium: 109mg

---

# Chocolate Lava Cake

**(Yields:** 2 servings / **Prep Time:** 15 minutes / **Cooking Time:** 9 minutes)

## Ingredients

- 2 ounces 70% dark chocolate
- 2 ounces unsalted butter

- 2 organic eggs
- 2 tablespoons powdered Erythritol plus more for dusting
- 1 tablespoon almond flour
- 6 fresh raspberries

## Instructions

1. Preheat the oven to 350 degrees F. Grease 2 ramekins.
2. In a microwave-safe bowl, add the chocolate, and butter and microwave on High for about 2 minutes or until melted, stirring after every 30 seconds.
3. Remove the bowl from microwave and stir until smooth.
4. Place the eggs in a bowl and with a wire whisk, beat well.
5. Add the chocolate mixture, Erythritol, and almond flour and mix until well combined.
6. Divide the mixture evenly into prepared ramekins.
7. Bake for about 9 minutes or until the top is set.
8. Remove the ramekins from oven and set aside for about 1-2 minutes.
9. Carefully, invert the cakes onto serving plates and dust with extra powdered Erythritol.
10. Garnish with fresh raspberries and serve.

## Nutrition Values (Per Serving)

- Calories: 436
- Net Carbs: 4.9g
- Carbohydrate: 11g
- Fiber: 6.1g
- Protein: 10.4g
- Fat: 25.2g
- Sugar: 1.4g
- Sodium: 232mg

# Hot Chocolate

(**Yields:** 2 servings / **Prep Time:** 10 minutes)

## Ingredients

- 2 ounces unsalted butter
- 4 tablespoons cacao powder
- 2 teaspoons powdered Erythritol
- ½ teaspoon organic vanilla extract
- 2 cups boiling water
- 2 tablespoons whipped cream

## Instructions

1. In a tall beaker, place all the ingredients except cream and with an immersion blender, blend for about 15-20 seconds or until a fine foam appears on top.
2. Transfer the hot chocolate into two mugs.
3. Top each mug with whipped cream and serve immediately.

### Nutrition Values (Per Serving)

- Calories: 269
- Net Carbs: 2g
- Carbohydrate: 4.3g
- Fiber: 2.3g
- Protein: 2.1g
- Fat: 29.1g
- Sugar: 0.2g
- Sodium: 169mg

## Chai Hot Chocolate

**(Yields:** 2 servings / **Prep Time:** 15 minutes / **Cooking Time:** 4 minutes)

### Ingredients

- 2 chai tea bags
- ½ cup hot water, divided
- 4 tablespoons cacao powder
- 1 cup unsweetened almond milk
- ½ teaspoon stevia powder
- 4 tablespoons cacao butter

### Instructions

1. Place the tea bags and 2 tablespoons of hot water in a bowl and let it steep for about 5 minutes.
2. In a small pan, add the cacao powder, and remaining water and beat well.
3. Add the almond milk and stir to combine.
4. Stir in the stevia and cacao butter.
5. Discard the tea bags and pour the tea into pan.
6. Cook for about 2-4 minutes or until butter is dissolved completely, stirring continuously.
7. Remove the pan from heat and transfer into serving cups.
8. Serve immediately.

### Nutrition Values (Per Serving)

- Calories: 161
- Net Carbs: 2.5g
- Carbohydrate: 6g
- Fiber: 3.5g
- Protein: 2.5g
- Fat: 17.3g
- Sugar: 0g
- Sodium: 90mg

## Butter Coffee

**(Yields:** 2 servings / **Prep Time:** 5 minutes / **Cooking Time:** 5 minutes)

### Ingredients

- 2 cups water
- 2 tablespoons ground coffee
- 1 tablespoon coconut oil
- 1 tablespoon butter

### Instructions

1. In a pan, add the water and coffee over medium heat and cook for about 5 minutes.
2. Through a strainer, strain the coffee into a blender.
3. Add the coconut oil, and butter and pulse until light and creamy.
4. Transfer into two mugs and serve immediately.

### Nutrition Values (Per Serving)

- Calories: 110
- Net Carbs: 0g
- Carbohydrate: 0g
- Fiber: 0g
- Protein: 0.1g
- Fat: 12.6g
- Sugar: 0g
- Sodium: 48mg

## Espresso Coffee

(**Yields:** 2 servings / **Prep Time:** 10 minutes)

### Ingredients

- 3-4 tablespoons Erythritol
- 2 tablespoons instant coffee powder
- 2 teaspoons water
- 2 cups hot unsweetened almond milk

### Instructions

1. In two coffee mugs, divide the Erythritol, coffee powder, and water and stir until well combined.
2. With a spoon, beat vigorously until frothy.
3. Pour hot milk over the whipped coffee paste in each mug and stir to combine.
4. Serve immediately.

### Nutrition Values (Per Serving)

- Calories: 40
- Net Carbs: 1g
- Carbohydrate: 2g
- Fiber: 1g
- Protein: 1g
- Fat: 3.5g
- Sugar: 0g
- Sodium: 180mg

## Cinnamon Cappuccino

(**Yields:** 4 servings / **Prep Time:** 10 minutes / **Cooking Time:** 10 minutes)

### Ingredients

- 2 cups unsweetened almond milk
- 1 cinnamon stick
- 2 cups strong coffee
- 3-4 tablespoons Erythritol
- Ground cinnamon, as required

## Instructions

1. In a pan, add the milk, and cinnamon stick and bring to a boil.
2. Adjust the heat to low and simmer for about 10 minutes.
3. Remove the pan from heat and discard the cinnamon stick.
4. Divide the coffee and Erythritol into 4 cups and stir to combine.
5. Now, pour the hot milk, raising it high.
6. Sprinkle with ground cinnamon and serve immediately.

## Nutrition Values (Per Serving)

- Calories: 22
- Net Carbs: 0.5g
- Carbohydrate: 1.1g
- Fiber: 0.6g
- Protein: 0.7g
- Fat: 1.8g
- Sugar: 0g
- Sodium: 92mg

---

# Gingerbread Latte

**(Yields:** 2 servings / **Prep Time:** 10 minutes)

## Ingredients

- ½ cup hot strong brewed coffee
- 1-2 tablespoons Erythritol
- ½ teaspoon ground cinnamon
- ½ teaspoon ground ginger
- ¼ teaspoon ground nutmeg
- ½ teaspoon organic vanilla extract
- 1¾ cups hot unsweetened almond milk

## Instructions

1. Add all the ingredients in a bowl except almond milk and beat until well combined.
2. Place the coffee mixture into two coffee mugs and top with the almond milk.
3. Spoon foam over the top and serve.

## Nutrition Values (Per Serving)

- Calories: 68
- Net Carbs: 2.2g
- Carbohydrate: 4.3g
- Fiber: 2.1g
- Protein: 1.8g
- Fat: 5.8g
- Sugar: 0.2g
- Sodium: 294mg

# Spiced Mocha

**(Yields:** 2 servings / **Prep Time:** 10 minutes/ **Total Cooking Time:** 5 minutes)

## Ingredients

- 1 cup unsweetened coconut milk
- 2 tablespoons Erythritol
- 2 tablespoons cacao powder
- 1 teaspoon organic vanilla extract
- ½ teaspoon ground cinnamon
- ¼ teaspoon ground cardamom
- Pinch of cayenne pepper
- 1½ cups brewed hot coffee
- 1 tablespoon MCT oil
- 3-4 tablespoons whipped cream

## Instructions

1. Place the coconut milk, Erythritol, cacao powder, vanilla extract and spices in a small pan and mix well.
2. Place the pan over medium heat and bring to a boil.
3. Cook for about 1 minute.
4. Remove from heat and stir in the coffee and MCT oil until well combined.
5. Transfer into 2 mugs and top each with the whipped cream.
6. Serve immediately.

## Nutrition Values (Per Serving)

- Calories: 161
- Net Carbs: 2.7g
- Carbohydrate: 5.1g
- Fiber: 2.4g
- Protein: 1.8g
- Fat: 17g
- Sugar: 0.3g
- Sodium: 12mg

---

# Spiced Tea

**(Yields:** 2 servings / **Prep Time:** 10 minutes / **Total Cooking Time:** 5 minutes)

## Ingredients

- 1 cup water
- 2 whole cloves
- 2 green cardamom pods
- Pinch of fennel seeds
- 2 black tea bags
- 1 cup unsweetened almond milk
- 12-14 drops liquid stevia

## Instructions

1. Place the water and spices in a small pan over medium-low heat and bring to a gentle simmer.
2. Add the tea bags and immediately, cover the pan for about 2 minutes.
3. Add the almond milk and bring to a boil.

4. Immediately, remove the pan from heat and set aside, covered for at least 1 minute.
5. Through a fine mesh strainer, strain the tea into serving cups.
6. Stir in the stevia and serve immediately.

## **Nutrition Values (Per Serving)**

- Calories: 21
- Net Carbs: 1.2g
- Carbohydrate: 1.2g
- Fiber: 0g
- Protein: 0.5g
- Fat: 1.8g
- Sugar: 0g
- Sodium: 90mg

## **Lemony Green Tea**

**(Yields:** 2 servings / **Prep Time:** 10 minutes)

## Ingredients

- 2½ cups boiling water
- 2 tablespoons loose leaf jasmine green tea
- 4 lemon slices
- 10-12 drops liquid stevia

## Instructions

1. In a pitcher, add all the ingredients and stir to combine.
2. Immediately, cover and steep for about 3-5 minutes.
3. Serve immediately.

## **Nutrition Values (Per Serving)**

- Calories: 1
- Net Carbs: 0.3g
- Carbohydrate: 0.4g
- Fiber: 0.1g
- Protein: 0g
- Fat: 0g
- Sugar: 0.1g
- Sodium: 0mg

## **Eggnog**

**(Yields:** 6 servings / **Prep Time:** 15 minutes / **Cooking Time:** 15 minutes)

## Ingredients

- 4 large organic eggs (whites and yolks separated)
- 2 cups heavy whipping cream
- 1 cup unsweetened almond milk
- ¾ cup powdered Erythritol
- ½ teaspoon organic vanilla extract
- ¼ teaspoon ground cinnamon
- ¼ teaspoon ground nutmeg

## Instructions

1. Place the egg yolks in a bowl and beat until smooth.
2. In a pan, place the heavy cream, almond milk, Erythritol and beaten egg yolks over medium-low heat and cook for about 10-15 minutes, stirring continuously.
3. Remove from heat and transfer the mixture into a heatproof bowl.
4. Add the vanilla extract, and spices and beat until well combined.
5. Set aside to cool completely.
6. Cover the bowl and refrigerate overnight.
7. In a bowl, add the egg whites and beat until soft peaks form.
8. Remove the bowl of eggnog from refrigerator and through a strainer, strain the mixture.
9. Add the whipped egg whites and stir to combine.
10. Transfer the eggnog into serving glasses and serve.

## Nutrition Values (Per Serving)

- Calories: 56
- Net Carbs: 0.6g
- Carbohydrate: 0.8g
- Fiber: 0.2g
- Protein: 4.4g
- Fat: 3.9g
- Sugar: 0.3g
- Sodium: 77mg

---

# Lemonade

**(Yields:** 2 servings / **Prep Time:** 10 minutes)

## Ingredients

- 2 cups water
- 2 tablespoons fresh lemon juice
- 2 tablespoons monk fruit sweetener
- Ice cubes, as required

## Instructions

1. In a pitcher, place all the ingredients and stir until well combined.
2. Fill the glasses with ice cubes and top with the lemon mixture.
3. Serve chilled.

## Nutrition Values (Per Serving)

- Calories: 4
- Net Carbs: 0.2g
- Carbohydrate: 0.3g
- Fiber: 0.1g
- Protein: 0.1g
- Fat: 0.1g
- Sugar: 0.3g
- Sodium: 3mg

**(Tip:** For better taste, make sure to use freshly squeezed lemon juice.)

# Ginger Lemonade

**(Yields:** 4 servings / **Prep Time:** 10 minutes)

## Ingredients

- 4-5 tablespoons fresh lemon juice
- 2 tablespoons fresh ginger, peeled and grated
- 1/3 cup powdered Erythritol
- 4 cups water
- Ice cubes, as required

## Instructions

1. In a pitcher, add the lemon juice, ginger, Erythritol, and water and stir until sweetener is dissolved.
2. Fill 4 serving glasses with ice cubes and top with the lemonade.
3. Serve chilled.

## Nutrition Values (Per Serving)

- Calories: 13
- Net Carbs: 1.8g
- Carbohydrate: 2.2g
- Fiber: 0.4g
- Protein: 0.4g
- Fat: 0.3g
- Sugar: 0.4g
- Sodium: 11mg

---

# Mint Green Tea

**(Yields:** 4 servings / **Prep Time:** 10 minutes)

## Ingredients

- 2½ cups boiling water
- 1 cup fresh mint leaves
- 4 green tea bags
- 2 teaspoons yacon syrup

## Instructions

1. In a pitcher, add the water, mint, and tea bags.
2. Cover and steep for about 5 minutes.

3. Refrigerate for at least 3 hours.
4. Discard the tea bags and divide the tea into serving glasses.
5. Add the yacon syrup and stir to combine.
6. Serve immediately.

## Nutrition Values (Per Serving)

- Calories: 14
- Net Carbs: 1.3g
- Carbohydrate: 2.9g
- Fiber: 1.6g
- Protein: 0.8g
- Fat: 0.2g
- Sugar: 0.6g
- Sodium: 8mg

---

# Creamy Iced Tea

**(Yields:** 2 servings / **Prep Time:** 10 minutes**)**

## Ingredients

- 2 black tea bags
- 1 cup boiling water
- 12-16 ice cubes
- ½ cup heavy cream
- 12-16 drops liquid stevia

## Instructions

1. In a pitcher, add the tea bags and water.
2. Immediately, cover and steep for about 4-5 minutes.
3. Divide the ice cubes into serving glasses.
4. Discard the tea bags and pour steeped tea into glasses over ice cubes.
5. Add the heavy cream and stir to combine.
6. Serve immediately.

## Nutrition Values (Per Serving)

- Calories: 104
- Net Carbs: 0.8g
- Carbohydrate: 0.8g
- Fiber: 0g
- Protein: 10.6g
- Fat: 11.1g
- Sugar: 0g
- Sodium: 11mg

# Iced Coffee

**(Yields:** 2 servings / **Prep Time:** 10 minutes)

## Ingredients

- 2 cups chilled brewed coffee
- 2 tablespoons heavy cream
- 1 tablespoon MCT oil
- 1 cup ice cubes
- 1 teaspoon organic vanilla extract
- ½ teaspoon liquid stevia
- ¼ teaspoon xanthan gum
- ¼ teaspoon ground cinnamon
- Pinch of sea salt

## Instructions

1. Place the coffee, heavy cream, MCT oil and 1 cup of ice cubes in a blender and pulse on high speed until well combined.
2. Add the remaining ingredients and pulse until smooth.
3. Add the desired amount of ice cubes into glasses.
4. Pour coffee over ice and serve.

## Nutrition Values (Per Serving)

- Calories: 118
- Net Carbs: 0.8g
- Carbohydrate: 2.6g
- Fiber: 1.8g
- Protein: 0.6g
- Fat: 12.6g
- Sugar: 0.3g
- Sodium: 163mg

# CHAPTER 10 | DRESSINGS, SAUCES & SEASONING

## Ranch Dressing

**(Yields:** 12 servings / **Prep Time:** 10 minutes)

### Ingredients

- 1 cup mayonnaise
- ½ cup sour cream
- ¼ cup unsweetened almond milk
- 2 teaspoons fresh lemon juice
- 2 teaspoons dried parsley
- 1 teaspoon dried chives
- 1 teaspoon dried dill
- ½ teaspoon garlic powder
- ½ teaspoon onion powder
- Salt and ground black pepper, as required

### Instructions

1. Add all the ingredients in a large bowl and beat until well combined.
2. Refrigerate to chill before serving.

### Nutrition Values (Per Serving)

- Calories: 99
- Net Carbs: 5.3g
- Carbohydrate: 5.4g
- Fiber: 0.1g
- Protein: 0.6g
- Fat: 8.6g
- Sugar: 1.4g
- Sodium: 60mg

---

## French Dressing

**(Yields:** 20 servings / **Prep Time:** 10 minutes)

### Ingredients

- 1 small yellow onion, roughly chopped
- 1½ cups olive oil
- 1 cup sugar-free ketchup
- ¾ cup Erythritol
- ½ cup balsamic vinegar
- 1 teaspoon fresh lemon juice
- 1 teaspoon paprika
- ½ teaspoon salt

### Instructions

1. Add all the ingredients in a blender and pulse until smooth.
2. Serve immediately.

## Nutrition Values (Per Serving)

- Calories: 144
- Net Carbs: 3.3g
- Carbohydrate: 3.5g
- Fiber: 0.2g
- Protein: 0.3g
- Fat: 15.2g
- Sugar: 2.9g
- Sodium: 61mg

---

# Caesar Dressing

**(Yields:** 16 servings / **Prep Time:** 10 minutes)

## Ingredients

- 1 organic egg yolk
- 2 tablespoons fresh lemon juice
- 1 tablespoon anchovy paste
- 2 teaspoons Dijon mustard
- 2 garlic cloves, peeled
- 1 tablespoon fresh oregano
- Salt and ground black pepper, as required
- ½ cup olive oil
- ½ cup Parmesan cheese, shredded

## Instructions

1. Place all the ingredients except oil and Parmesan in a blender and pulse until smooth.
2. While the motor is running gradually, add the oil and pulse until smooth.
3. Add the Parmesan cheese and pulse for about 20 seconds.
4. Serve immediately.

## Nutrition Values (Per Serving)

- Calories: 72
- Net Carbs: 0.3g
- Carbohydrate: 0.5g
- Fiber: 0.2g
- Protein: 1.3g
- Fat: 8.7g
- Sugar: 0.1g
- Sodium: 121mg

---

# Yogurt Dressing

**(Yields:** 8 servings / **Prep Time:** 10 minutes)

## Ingredients

- 1 (8-ounces) container plain Greek yogurt
- 2 teaspoons fresh lemon juice
- 1 teaspoon fresh chives, chopped
- 1 teaspoon fresh parsley, chopped
- 1 teaspoon Dijon mustard

## Instructions

1. Place the yogurt and lemon juice in a bowl and beat until well combined and smooth.
2. Now, place the remaining ingredients and stir until well combined.
3. Refrigerate before serving.

## Nutrition Values (Per Serving)

- Calories: 21
- Net Carbs: 2.1g
- Carbohydrate: 2.1g
- Fiber: 0g
- Protein: 1.7g
- Fat: 0.4g
- Sugar: 2g
- Sodium: 27mg

---

# Blue Cheese Dressing

**(Yields:** 24 servings / **Prep Time:** 10 minutes)

## Ingredients

- 1 cup blue cheese, crumbled
- 1 cup sour cream
- 1 cup mayonnaise
- 2-4 drops liquid stevia
- 2 teaspoons fresh lemon juice
- 2 teaspoons Worcestershire sauce
- 1 teaspoon hot pepper sauce
- 2 tablespoons fresh parsley, chopped
- Salt and ground black pepper, as required

## Instructions

1. Add all the ingredients in a large bowl and beat until well combined.
2. Refrigerate to chill before serving.

## Nutrition Values (Per Serving)

- Calories: 101
- Net Carbs: 0.7g
- Carbohydrate: 0.7g
- Fiber: 0g
- Protein: 1.5g
- Fat: 10.3g
- Sugar: 0.1g
- Sodium: 156mg

# Olives & Feta Dressing

**(Yields:** 16 servings / **Prep Time:** 10 minutes)

## Ingredients

- 3 tablespoons feta cheese, crumbled
- 3 tablespoons kalamata olives, pitted and chopped
- 2 tablespoons yellow onion, chopped
- 1 garlic clove, chopped
- 6-8 drops liquid stevia
- 1 tablespoon Dijon mustard
- 3 tablespoons fresh lemon juice
- 3 tablespoons olive oil
- 1 teaspoon dried oregano, crushed
- Salt and ground black pepper, as required

## Instructions

1. Add all the ingredients in a blender and pulse until smooth.
2. Serve immediately.

## Nutrition Values (Per Serving)

- Calories: 31
- Net Carbs: 0.3g
- Carbohydrate: 0.5g
- Fiber: 0.2g
- Protein: 0.4g
- Fat: 3.2g
- Sugar: 0.2g
- Sodium: 57mg

---

# Creamy Mustard Dressing

**(Yields:** 8 servings / **Prep Time:** 10 minutes)

## Ingredients

- ½ cup sour cream
- ¼ cup water
- ¼ cup Dijon mustard
- 1 tablespoon organic apple cider vinegar
- 1 tablespoon granulated Erythritol

## Instructions

1. Add all the ingredients in a large bowl and beat until well combined.
2. Serve immediately.

## Nutrition Values (Per Serving)

- Calories: 36
- Net Carbs: 0.8g
- Carbohydrate: 1.1g
- Fiber: 0.3g
- Protein: 0.8g
- Fat: 3.3g
- Sugar: 0.1g
- Sodium: 97mg

# Sunflower Seeds Dressing

**(Yields:** 5 servings / **Prep Time:** 1 minutes)

## Ingredients

- ½ cup sunflower seeds
- 1/3 cup organic apple cider vinegar
- ½ cup water
- 1 tablespoon Dijon mustard
- 1 teaspoon ground turmeric
- Salt and ground black pepper, as required
- ¼ cup olive oil

## Instructions

1. Add all the ingredients except oil in a blender and pulse until smooth.
2. While the motor is running gradually, add the oil and pulse until smooth.
3. Serve immediately.

## Nutrition Values (Per Serving)

- Calories: 120
- Net Carbs: 0.9g
- Carbohydrate: 1.5g
- Fiber: 0.6g
- Protein: 1.1g
- Fat: 12.6g
- Sugar: 0.2g
- Sodium: 69mg

---

# Italian Dressing

**(Yields:** 12 servings / **Prep Time:** 10 minutes)

## Ingredients

- 1 cup olive oil
- ½ cup balsamic vinegar
- 1 teaspoon dried basil
- ½ teaspoon dried oregano
- 1/8 teaspoon dried marjoram
- Salt and ground black pepper, as required
- 2 tablespoons Pecorino Romano cheese, grated finely
- 1 tablespoon garlic, minced

## Instructions

1. Place the oil, vinegar, dried herbs, salt, and black pepper in a blender and pulse until well combined.
2. Place the dressing into a bowl and stir in the cheese and garlic.
3. Serve.

### Nutrition Values (Per Serving)

- Calories: 152
- Net Carbs: 0.4g
- Carbohydrate: 0.4g
- Fiber: 0g
- Protein: 0.4g
- Fat: 17.1g
- Sugar: 0.1g
- Sodium: 36mg

---

## Raspberry Dressing

**(Yields:** 10 servings / **Prep Time:** 10 minutes)

### Ingredients

- ½ cup olive oil
- ¼ cup MCT oil
- ¼ cup organic apple cider vinegar
- 2 tablespoons Dijon mustard
- 1½ teaspoons fresh tarragon leaves, chopped
- ¼ teaspoon Erythritol
- Pinch of salt
- ½ cup fresh raspberries, mashed

### Instructions

1. Place all the ingredients except raspberries in a bowl and beat until smooth.
2. Transfer the mixture into a bowl.
3. Now, add the mashed raspberries and stir to combine well.
4. Serve immediately.

### Nutrition Values (Per Serving)

- Calories: 133
- Net Carbs: 0.5g
- Carbohydrate: 1g
- Fiber: 0.5g
- Protein: 0.2g
- Fat: 15.9g
- Sugar: 0.2g
- Sodium: 51mg

---

## Cranberry Sauce

**(Yields:** 6 servings / **Prep Time:** 10 minutes / **Cooking Time:** 15 minutes)

### Ingredients

- 12 ounces fresh cranberries
- 1 cup powdered Erythritol
- ¾ cup water
- 1 teaspoon fresh lemon zest, grated
- ½ teaspoon organic vanilla extract

## Instructions

1. Place the cranberries, water, Erythritol and lemon zest in a medium pan and mix well.
2. Place the pan over medium heat and bring to a boil.
3. Adjust the heat to low and simmer for about 12-15 minutes, stirring frequently.
4. Remove the pan from heat and mix in the vanilla extract.
5. Set aside at room temperature to cool completely.
6. Transfer the sauce into a bowl and refrigerate to chill before serving.

## Nutrition Values (Per Serving)

- Calories: 32
- Net Carbs: 3.1g
- Carbohydrate: 5.2g
- Fiber: 2.1g
- Protein: 0g
- Fat: 0g
- Sugar: 2.1g
- Sodium: 160mg

---

# Ketchup

**(Yields:** 12 servings / **Prep Time:** 10 minutes / **Cooking Time:** 30 minutes)

## Ingredients

- 6 ounces sugar-free tomato paste
- 1 cup water
- ¼ cup powdered Erythritol
- 3 tablespoons balsamic vinegar
- ½ teaspoon garlic powder
- ½ teaspoon onion powder
- ¼ teaspoon paprika
- 1/8 teaspoon ground cloves
- 1/8 tsp mustard powder
- Salt, as required

## Instructions

1. Add all the ingredients in a small pan and beat until smooth.
2. Now, place the pan over medium heat and bring to a gentle simmer, stirring continuously.
3. Adjust the heat to low and simmer, covered for about 30 minutes or until desired thickness, stirring occasionally.
4. Remove the pan from heat and let it cool completely before serving.
5. You can preserve this ketchup in the refrigerator by placing in an airtight container.

## Nutrition Values (Per Serving)

- Calories: 13
- Net Carbs: 2.3g
- Carbohydrate: 2.9g
- Fiber: 0.6g

- Protein: 0.7g
- Fat: 0.1g
- Sugar: 1.8g
- Sodium: 26mg

**(Note:** For the best consistency, puree the ketchup in a high-speed blender until smooth.)

## Cilantro Sauce

**(Yields:** 6 servings / **Prep Time:** 10 minutes)

### Ingredients

- ½ cup plain Greek yogurt
- ½ cup fresh cilantro, chopped
- 6 garlic cloves, peeled
- 1 jalapeño pepper, chopped
- Salt, as required
- ¼ cup water

### Instructions

1. Add all the ingredients in a blender and pulse until smooth.
2. Transfer the sauce into a bowl and set aside for about 15-20 minutes before serving.

### Nutrition Values (Per Serving)

- Calories: 20
- Net Carbs: 2.4g
- Carbohydrate: 2.6g
- Fiber: 0.2g
- Protein: 1.4g
- Fat: 0.3g
- Sugar: 1.6g
- Sodium: 43mg

## Avocado Sauce

**(Yields:** 8 servings / **Prep Time:** 15 minutes)

### Ingredients

- 2 avocados, peeled, pitted and chopped
- ½ cup yellow onion, chopped
- 1 cup fresh cilantro leaves
- 2 garlic cloves, chopped
- 1 jalapeño pepper, chopped
- 1 cup homemade vegetable broth
- 2 tablespoons fresh lemon juice
- 2 teaspoons balsamic vinegar
- 1 teaspoon ground cumin
- Pinch of cayenne pepper
- Salt, as required

## Instructions

1. Add all the ingredients in a blender and pulse until smooth.
2. Serve immediately.

## Nutrition Values (Per Serving)

- Calories: 115
- Net Carbs: 2.1g
- Carbohydrate: 5.8g
- Fiber: 3.7g
- Protein: 1.8g
- Fat: 10.1g
- Sugar: 0.8g
- Sodium: 120mg

---

# Herbed Capers Sauce

**(Yields:** 4 servings / **Prep Time:** 10 minutes)

## Ingredients

- ½ cup fresh parsley, finely chopped
- 3 tablespoons fresh basil, finely chopped
- 2 garlic cloves, crushed
- 1 tablespoon fresh lemon juice
- 2 tablespoons small capers
- ¾ cup olive oil
- Salt and ground black pepper, as required

## Instructions

1. Add all the ingredients into a shallow bowl and with an immersion blender, blend until the desired consistency is achieved.
2. Serve immediately.

## Nutrition Values (Per Serving)

- Calories: 331
- Net Carbs: 0.8g
- Carbohydrate: 1.3g
- Fiber: 0.5g
- Protein: 0.5g
- Fat: 38g
- Sugar: 0.2g
- Sodium: 172mg

---

# Basil Pesto

**(Yields:** 6 servings / **Prep Time:** 10 minutes)

## Ingredients

- 2 cups fresh basil
- 4 garlic cloves, peeled
- 2/3 cup Parmesan cheese, grated
- 1/3 cup pine nuts

- ½ cup olive oil
- Salt and ground black pepper, as required

## Instructions

1. Place the basil, garlic, Parmesan cheese and pine nuts in a food processor and pulse until a chunky mixture is formed.
2. While the motor is running gradually, add the oil and pulse until smooth.
3. Now, add the salt, and black pepper and pulse until well combined.
4. Serve immediately.

## Nutrition Values (Per Serving)

- Calories: 232
- Net Carbs: 1.4g
- Carbohydrate: 1.9g
- Fiber: 0.5g
- Protein: 5g
- Fat: 24.2g
- Sugar: 0.3g
- Sodium: 104mg

---

# Veggie Hummus

**(Yields:** 8 servings / **Prep Time:** 10 minutes)

## Ingredients

- 2½ tablespoons olive oil, divided
- 1 cup zucchini, peeled and chopped
- ¾ cup pumpkin puree
- ¼ cup tahini
- 2 tablespoons fresh lemon juice
- 1 teaspoon ground cumin
- 1 teaspoon garlic powder
- ½ teaspoon smoked paprika
- Salt, as required

## Instructions

1. Place 2 tablespoons of oil and the remaining ingredients in a blender and pulse until smooth.
2. Place the hummus into a bowl and drizzle with remaining oil.
3. Serve immediately.

## Nutrition Values (Per Serving)

- Calories: 96
- Net Carbs: 2.7g
- Carbohydrate: 4.4g
- Fiber: 1.7g
- Protein: 1.9g
- Fat: 8.6g
- Sugar: 1.2g
- Sodium: 32mg

# Tzatziki

**(Yields:** 12 servings / **Prep Time:** 10 minutes)

## Ingredients

- 1 large English cucumber, peeled and grated
- Salt, as required
- 2 cups plain Greek yogurt
- 1 tablespoon fresh lemon juice
- 4 garlic cloves, minced
- 1 tablespoon fresh mint leaves, chopped
- 2 tablespoons fresh dill, chopped
- Pinch of cayenne pepper
- Freshly ground black pepper, as required

## Instructions

1. Arrange a colander in the sink.
2. Place the cucumber into colander and sprinkle with salt.
3. Let it drain for about 10-15 minutes.
4. With your hands, squeeze the cucumber well.
5. Place the cucumber and remaining ingredients in a large bowl and stir to combine.
6. Cover the bowl and refrigerate to chill for at least 4-8 hours before serving.

## Nutrition Values (Per Serving)

- Calories: 36
- Net Carbs: 4.2g
- Carbohydrate: 4.5g
- Fiber: 0.3g
- Protein: 2.7g
- Fat: 0.6g
- Sugar: 3.3g
- Sodium: 42mg

---

# Baba Ghanoush

**(Yields:** 8 servings / **Prep Time:** 15 minutes / **Cooking Time:** 35 minutes)

## Ingredients

- 2 large eggplants
- 3 teaspoons olive oil
- 2 garlic cloves, chopped
- 2 tablespoons tahini
- 2 tablespoons fresh lemon juice
- 1 teaspoon ground cumin
- Salt and ground black pepper, as required
- 1 tablespoon fresh parsley leaves

## Instructions

1. Preheat the oven to 400 degrees F. Grease a baking dish.
2. Arrange the eggplants into prepared baking dish in a single layer.
3. Bake for about 35 minutes.

4. Remove the eggplants from oven and immediately, place into a bowl of cold water to cool slightly.
5. Now, peel off the skin of eggplants.
6. Place the eggplants, 2 teaspoons of oil and remaining ingredients except parsley and pulse until smooth.
7. Place the mixture into a serving bowl and refrigerate to chill before serving.
8. Drizzle with the remaining oil and serve with garnishing of fresh parsley.

## **Nutrition Values (Per Serving)**

- Calories: 75
- Net Carbs: 4g
- Carbohydrate: 9.3g
- Fiber: 5.3g
- Protein: 2.1g
- Fat: 4.1g
- Sugar: 4.2g
- Sodium: 28mg

---

# **Salsa Verde**

(**Yields:** 10 servings / **Prep Time:** 15 minutes / **Cooking Time:** 40 minutes)

## **Ingredients**

- 2 pounds medium tomatillos, husks removed and halved
- 2 large yellow onions, roughly chopped
- 6 garlic cloves, peeled and halved
- 2 Serrano peppers, seeded and chopped
- ¼ cup olive oil
- 1/3-½ cup water
- ½ cup fresh cilantro, chopped
- 2 tablespoons fresh lime juice
- Pinch of salt

## **Instructions**

1. Preheat the oven to 425 degrees F.
2. In a large bowl, add the tomatillos, onions, garlic, peppers, and oil and toss to coat well.
3. Place the mixture onto 2 (15x10x1-inch) baking sheets and spread in an even layer.
4. Roast for about 35-40 minutes, stirring occasionally.
5. Remove both baking sheets from the oven and set aside to cool slightly.
6. Place the tomatillo mixture and enough water in a food processor and pulse until smooth.
7. Now, add the remaining ingredients and pulse until just combined.
8. Transfer the mixture into a bowl and refrigerate to chill before serving.

### **Nutrition Values (Per Serving)**

- Calories: 84
- Net Carbs: 5.8g
- Carbohydrate: 8.1g
- Fiber: 2.3g
- Protein: 1.3g
- Fat: 6g
- Sugar: 1g
- Sodium: 18mg

---

## Pizza Sauce

**(Yields:** 8 servings / **Prep Time:** 15 minutes / **Cooking Time:** 45 minutes)

### Ingredients

- 2 tablespoons olive oil
- 2 anchovy fillets
- 2 tablespoons fresh oregano leaves, finely chopped
- 3 garlic cloves, minced
- ½ teaspoon dried oregano, crushed
- ½ teaspoon red pepper flakes, crushed
- 1 (28-ounces) can whole peeled tomatoes, crushed
- ½ teaspoon Erythritol
- Salt, as required
- Pinch of freshly ground black pepper
- Pinch of organic baking powder

### Instructions

1. Heat the olive oil in a medium pan over medium-low heat and cook the anchovy fillets for about 1 minute, stirring occasionally.
2. Stir in the fresh oregano, garlic, dried oregano, and red pepper flakes and sauté for about 2-3 minutes.
3. Add the remaining ingredients except baking powder and bring to a gentle simmer.
4. Reduce the heat to low and simmer for about 35-40 minutes, stirring occasionally.
5. Stir in the baking powder and remove from heat.
6. Set aside at room temperature to cool completely before serving.
7. You can preserve this sauce in refrigerator by placing into an airtight container.

### **Nutrition Values (Per Serving)**

- Calories: 56
- Net Carbs: 3.4g
- Carbohydrate: 5.1g
- Fiber: 1.7g
- Protein: 1.4g
- Fat: 4g
- Sugar: 2.7g
- Sodium: 61mg

# Marinara Sauce

**(Yields:** 12 servings / **Prep Time:** 10 minutes / **Total Cooking Time:** 5 minutes)

## Ingredients

- 2 tablespoons olive oil
- 1 garlic clove
- 2 teaspoons onion flakes
- 2 teaspoons fresh thyme, finely chopped
- 2 teaspoons fresh oregano, finely chopped
- 24 ounces tomato puree
- 1 tablespoon balsamic vinegar
- 2 teaspoons Erythritol
- Salt and ground black pepper, as required
- 2 tablespoons fresh parsley, finely chopped

## Instructions

1. Heat the olive oil in a medium pan over medium-low heat and sauté the garlic, onion flakes, thyme and oregano for about 3 minutes.
2. Stir in the tomato puree, vinegar, Erythritol, salt, and black pepper and bring to a gentle simmer.
3. Remove the pan of sauce from heat and stir in the parsley.
4. Set aside at room temperature to cool completely before serving.
5. You can preserve this sauce in refrigerator by placing into an airtight container.

## Nutrition Values (Per Serving)

- Calories: 36
- Net Carbs: 3.6g
- Carbohydrate: 4.7g
- Fiber: 1.1g
- Protein: 0.9g
- Fat: 2g
- Sugar: 2.3g
- Sodium: 168mg

---

# BBQ Sauce

**(Yields:** 20 servings / **Prep Time:** 15 minutes / **Cooking Time:** 20 minutes)

## Ingredients

- 2½ (6-ounces) cans tomato paste
- ½ cup organic apple cider vinegar
- 1/3 cup powdered Erythritol
- 2 tablespoons Worcestershire sauce
- 1 tablespoon liquid hickory smoke
- 2 teaspoons smoked paprika
- 1 teaspoon garlic powder
- ½ teaspoon onion powder
- Salt, as required
- ¼ teaspoon red chili powder
- ¼ teaspoon cayenne pepper
- 1½ cups water

## Instructions

1. Add all the ingredients except water in a pan and beat until well combined.
2. Add 1 cup of water and beat until combined.
3. Add the remaining water and beat until well combined.
4. Place the pan over medium-high heat and bring to a gentle boil.
5. Adjust the heat to medium-low and simmer, uncovered for about 20 minutes, stirring frequently.
6. Remove from the heat and set aside to cool slightly before serving.
7. You can preserve this sauce in refrigerator by placing into an airtight container.

## Nutrition Values (Per Serving)

- Calories: 22
- Net Carbs: 3.7g
- Carbohydrate: 4.7g
- Fiber: 1g
- Protein: 1g
- Fat: 0.1g
- Sugar: 3g
- Sodium: 85mg

---

# Enchilada Sauce

**(Yields:** 6 servings / **Prep Time:** 10 minutes / **Total Cooking Time:** 10 minutes)

## Ingredients

- 3 ounces salted butter
- 1½ tablespoons Erythritol
- 2 teaspoons dried oregano
- 3 teaspoons ground cumin
- 2 teaspoons ground coriander
- 2 teaspoons onion powder
- ¼ teaspoon cayenne pepper
- Salt and ground black pepper, as required
- 12 ounces tomato puree

## Instructions

1. Melt the butter in a medium pan over medium heat and sauté all the ingredients except tomato puree for about 3 minutes.
2. Add the tomato puree and simmer for about 5 minutes.
3. Remove the pan from heat and let it cool slightly before serving.
4. You can preserve this sauce in the refrigerator by placing into an airtight container.

## Nutrition Values (Per Serving)

- Calories: 132
- Net Carbs: 5.1g
- Carbohydrate: 6.6g
- Fiber: 1.5g
- Protein: 1.4g
- Fat: 11.9g
- Sugar: 3.1g
- Sodium: 127mg

**(Note:** You can add a little water, if you prefer a thinner sauce.)

# Teriyaki Sauce

**(Yields:** 8 servings / **Prep Time:** 10 minutes / **Total Cooking Time:** 15 minutes)

## Ingredients

- ½ cup low-sodium soy sauce
- 1 cup water
- 2 tablespoons organic apple cider vinegar
- ¼ cup Erythritol
- 1 tablespoon sesame oil
- ½ teaspoon ginger powder
- 2 teaspoons garlic powder
- ½ teaspoon xanthan gum
- 2 teaspoons sesame seeds

## Instructions

1. Place all the ingredient except xanthan gum and sesame seeds in a small pan and mix well.
2. Now, place the pan over medium heat and bring to a boil.
3. Sprinkle with the xanthan gum and beat until well combined.
4. Cook for about 8-10 minutes or until the sauce becomes thick.
5. Remove the pan from heat and mix in the sesame seeds.
6. Serve hot.
7. You can preserve this cooled sauce in the refrigerator by placing into an airtight container.

## Nutrition Values (Per Serving)

- Calories: 29
- Net Carbs: 1.6g
- Carbohydrate: 2g
- Fiber: 0.4g
- Protein: 1.3g
- Fat: 2.1g
- Sugar: 1.2g
- Sodium: 886mg

---

# Hoisin Sauce

**(Yields:** 8 servings / **Prep Time:** 10 minutes)

## Ingredients

- 4 tablespoons low-sodium soy sauce
- 2 tablespoons natural peanut butter
- 1 tablespoon Erythritol
- 2 teaspoons balsamic vinegar
- 2 teaspoons sesame oil
- 1 teaspoon Sriracha
- 1 garlic clove, peeled
- Ground black pepper, as required

## Instructions

1. Add all the ingredients in a food processor and pulse until smooth.
2. You can preserve this sauce in the refrigerator by placing into an airtight container.

### **Nutrition Values (Per Serving)**

- Calories: 39
- Net Carbs: 1.2g
- Carbohydrate: 1.5g
- Fiber: 0.3g
- Protein: 1.8g
- Fat: 3.1g
- Sugar: 0.8g
- Sodium: 445mg

---

## **Hot Sauce**

(**Yields:** 40 servings / **Prep Time:** 15 minutes / **Cooking Time:** 15 minutes)

## **Ingredients**

- 1 tablespoon olive oil
- 1 cup carrot, peeled and chopped
- ½ cup yellow onion, chopped
- 5 garlic cloves, minced
- 6 habanero peppers, stemmed
- 1 tomato, chopped
- 1 tablespoon fresh lemon zest
- ¼ cup fresh lemon juice
- ¼ cup balsamic vinegar
- ¼ cup water
- Salt and ground black pepper, as required

## **Instructions**

1. Heat the oil in a large pan over medium heat and cook the carrot, onion and garlic for about 8-10 minutes, stirring frequently.
2. Remove the pan from heat and let it cool slightly.
3. Place the onion mixture and remaining ingredients in a food processor and pulse until smooth.
4. Return the mixture into the same pan over medium-low heat and simmer for about 3-5 minutes, stirring occasionally.
5. Remove the pan from heat and let it cool completely.
6. You can preserve this sauce in the refrigerator by placing into an airtight container.

## **Nutrition Values (Per Serving)**

- Calories: 9
- Net Carbs: 1g
- Carbohydrate: 1.3g
- Fiber: 0.3g
- Protein: 0.2g
- Fat: 0.4g
- Sugar: 0.7g
- Sodium: 7mg

# Worcestershire Sauce

**(Yields:** 10 servings / **Prep Time:** 5 minutes / **Total Cooking Time:** 5 minutes)

## Ingredients

- ½ cup organic apple cider vinegar
- 2 tablespoons low-sodium soy sauce
- 2 tablespoons water
- ¼ teaspoon ground mustard
- ¼ teaspoon ground ginger
- ¼ teaspoon garlic powder
- ¼ teaspoon onion powder
- 1/8 teaspoon ground cinnamon
- 1/8 teaspoon ground black pepper

## Instructions

1. Add all the ingredients in a small pan and mix well.
2. Now, place the pan over medium heat and bring to a boil.
3. Adjust the heat to low and simmer for about 1-2 minutes.
4. Remove the pan from heat and let it cool completely.
5. You can preserve this sauce in refrigerator by placing into an airtight container.

## Nutrition Values (Per Serving)

- Calories: 5
- Net Carbs: 0.4g
- Carbohydrate: 0.5g
- Fiber: 0.1g
- Protein: 0.2g
- Fat: 0g
- Sugar: 0.3g
- Sodium: 177mg

---

# Almond Butter

**(Yields:** 6 servings / **Prep Time:** 15 minutes / **Cooking Time:** 15 minutes)

## Ingredients

- 2¼ cups raw almonds
- 1 tablespoon coconut oil
- ¾ teaspoon salt
- 4-6 drops liquid stevia
- ½ teaspoon ground cinnamon

## Instructions

1. Preheat the oven to 325 degrees F.
2. Arrange the almonds onto a rimmed baking sheet in an even layer.
3. Bake for about 12-15 minutes.
4. Remove the almonds from oven and let them cool completely.

5. In a food processor, fitted with metal blade, place the almonds and pulse until a fine meal forms.
6. Add the coconut oil, and salt and pulse for about 6-9 minutes.
7. Add the stevia, and cinnamon and pulse for about 1-2 minutes.
8. You can preserve this almond butter in refrigerator by placing into an airtight container.

## Nutrition Values (Per Serving)

- Calories: 226
- Net Carbs: 3.2g
- Carbohydrate: 7.8g
- Fiber: 4.6g
- Protein: 7.6g
- Fat: 20.1g
- Sugar: 1.5g
- Sodium: 291mg

---

# Mayonnaise

**(Yields:** 10 servings / **Prep Time:** 10 minutes)

## Ingredients

- 2 organic egg yolks
- 3 teaspoons fresh lemon juice, divided
- 1 teaspoon mustard
- ½ cup coconut oil, melted
- ½ cup olive oil
- Salt and ground black pepper, as required (optional)

## Instructions

1. Place the egg yolks, 1 teaspoon of lemon juice, and mustard in a blender and pulse until combined.
2. While the motor is running gradually, add both oils and pulse until a thick mixture forms.
3. Add the remaining lemon juice, salt, and black pepper and pulse until well combined.
4. You can preserve this mayonnaise in refrigerator by placing into an airtight container.

## Nutrition Values (Per Serving)

- Calories: 193
- Net Carbs: 0.2g
- Carbohydrate: 0.3g
- Fiber: 0.1g
- Protein: 0.6g
- Fat: 22g
- Sugar: 0.1g
- Sodium: 17mg

**(Note:** If the mayonnaise seems too thin, slowly add more oils while the motor is running until thick.)

# Seasoned Salt

**(Yields:** 18 servings / **Prep Time:** 5 minutes)

## Ingredients

- ¼ cup kosher salt
- ½ teaspoon onion powder
- 1 teaspoon garlic powder
- 1 teaspoon paprika
- ½ teaspoon ground red pepper
- 4 teaspoons freshly ground black pepper

## Instructions

1. Add all the ingredients in a bowl and stir to combine.
2. Transfer into an airtight jar to preserve.

## Nutrition Values (Per Serving)

- Calories: 2
- Net Carbs: 0.4g
- Carbohydrate: 0.6g
- Fiber: 0.2g
- Protein: 0.1g
- Fat: 0.1g
- Sugar: 0.1g
- Sodium: 1500mg

---

# Poultry Seasoning

**(Yields:** 10 servings / **Prep Time:** 5 minutes)

## Ingredients

- 2 teaspoons dried sage, crushed finely
- 1 teaspoon dried marjoram, crushed finely
- ¾ teaspoon dried rosemary, crushed finely
- 1½ teaspoons dried thyme, crushed finely
- ½ teaspoon ground nutmeg
- ½ teaspoon ground black pepper

## Instructions

1. Add all the ingredients in a bowl and stir to combine.
2. Transfer into an airtight jar to preserve.

## Nutrition Values (Per Serving)

- Calories: 2
- Net Carbs: 0.2g
- Carbohydrate: 0.4g
- Fiber: 0.2g
- Protein: 0.1g
- Fat: 0.1g
- Sugar: 0g
- Sodium: 0mg

# Taco Seasoning

**(Yields:** 12 servings / **Prep Time:** 5 minutes)

## Ingredients

- ½ teaspoon dried oregano, crushed
- ½ teaspoon ground cumin
- 2 teaspoons hot chili powder
- 1½ teaspoons paprika
- Pinch of red pepper flakes, crushed
- Pinch of cayenne pepper
- ¼ teaspoon ground black pepper
- 1 teaspoon onion powder
- ½ teaspoon garlic powder
- ½ teaspoon sea salt

## Instructions

1. Add all the ingredients in a bowl and stir to combine.
2. Transfer into an airtight jar to preserve.

## Nutrition Values (Per Serving)

- Calories: 4
- Net Carbs: 0.5g
- Carbohydrate: 0.8g
- Fiber: 0.3g
- Protein: 0.2g
- Fat: 0.1g
- Sugar: 0.2g
- Sodium: 83mg

---

# Pumpkin Pie Spice

**(Yields:** 3 servings / **Prep Time:** 5 minutes)

## Ingredients

- 1 teaspoon ground cinnamon
- ¼ teaspoon ground ginger
- ¼ teaspoon ground nutmeg
- 1/8 teaspoon ground cloves

## Instructions

1. Add all the ingredients in a bowl and stir to combine.
2. Transfer into an airtight jar to preserve.

## Nutrition Values (Per Serving)

- Calories: 4
- Net Carbs: 0.4g
- Carbohydrate: 0.9g
- Fiber: 0.5g
- Protein: 0.1g
- Fat: 0.1g
- Sugar: 0.1g
- Sodium: 0mg

# Curry Powder

(**Yields:** 20 servings / **Prep Time:** 10 minutes / **Cooking Time:** 10 minutes)

## Ingredients

- ¼ cup coriander seeds
- 2 tablespoons mustard seeds
- 2 tablespoons cumin seeds
- 2 tablespoons anise seeds
- 1 tablespoon whole allspice berries
- 1 tablespoon fenugreek seeds
- 5 tablespoons ground turmeric

## Instructions

1. In a large nonstick frying pan, place all the spices except turmeric over medium heat and cook for about 9-10 minutes or until toasted completely, stirring continuously.
2. Remove the frying pan from heat and set aside to cool.
3. In a spice grinder, add the toasted spices, and turmeric and grind until a fine powder forms.
4. Transfer into an airtight jar to preserve.

## Nutrition Values (Per Serving)

- Calories: 19
- Net Carbs: 0.6g
- Carbohydrate: 2.4g
- Fiber: 1.8g
- Protein: 0.8g
- Fat: 0.8g
- Sugar: 0.1g
- Sodium: 2mg

# CHAPTER 11 | GLUTEN & DAIRY-FREE, VEGAN

## Fresh Strawberry Juice

**(Yields:** 3 servings / **Prep Time:** 10 minutes)

### Ingredients

- 2 cups fresh strawberries, hulled and sliced
- 2 cups chilled water
- 1 teaspoon fresh lime juice
- 1-2 drops liquid stevia
- Pinch of salt

### Instructions

1. Add all the ingredients in a blender and pulse until finely pureed.
2. Through a cheesecloth-lined strainer, strain the juice and transfer into serving glasses.
3. Serve immediately.

### Nutrition Values (Per Serving)

- Calories: 31
- Net Carbs: 5.5g
- Carbohydrate: 7.4g
- Fiber: 1.9g
- Protein: 0.6g
- Fat: 0.3g
- Sugar: 4g
- Sodium: 51mg

---

## Overnight Porridge

**(Yields:** 2 servings / **Prep Time:** 10 minutes)

### Ingredients

- 2/3 cup plus ¼ cup unsweetened coconut milk, divided
- ½ cup hemp hearts
- 1 tablespoon chia seed
- 3-4 drops liquid stevia
- ½ teaspoon organic vanilla extract
- Pinch of salt

### Instructions

1. Place 2/3 cup of coconut milk, hemp hearts, chia seed, stevia, vanilla extract and salt in a larger airtight container and stir until well combined.
2. Cover the container tightly and refrigerate overnight.
3. Just before serving, add the remaining coconut milk and stir to combine.
4. Serve immediately.

### Nutrition Values (Per Serving)

- Calories: 503
- Net Carbs: 3.8g
- Carbohydrate: 11.5g
- Fiber: 7.7g
- Protein: 16.g
- Fat: 45.4g
- Sugar: 5g
- Sodium: 99mg

---

## Mocha Cereal

**(Yields:** 4 servings / **Prep Time:** 15 minutes / **Cooking Time:** 30 minutes)

### Ingredients

- ½ cup golden flax seeds meal
- ¼ cup hemp seeds, hulled
- ¼ cup hazelnut meal
- 1 tablespoon cacao powder
- 3 packets stevia
- 1 tablespoon ground cinnamon
- ½ cup cold brewed coffee
- 1 tablespoon coconut oil

### Instructions

1. Preheat the oven to 300 degrees F. Line a large baking sheet with a parchment paper.
2. Place the flax seeds meal, hemp seeds, hazelnut meal, cacao powder and stevia in a high-speed blender and pulse until well combined.
3. Add the cinnamon, coffee, and coconut oil and pulse for about 30 more seconds.
4. Place the mocha mixture onto prepared baking sheet and with the back of a spoon, press firmly to smooth the top surface.
5. Bake for about 15 minutes.
6. Now, reduce the temperature of oven to 250 degrees F and bake for about 15 more minutes.
7. Remove the baking sheet from oven and immediately with a pizza cutter, cut the mixture into bite-sized pieces.
8. Turn off the oven and place baking sheet inside oven for at least 1 hour.
9. Remove the baking sheet from oven and let the cereal cool completely before serving.
10. Serve with your favorite non-dairy milk.

### Nutrition Values (Per Serving)

- Calories: 205
- Net Carbs: 2.9g
- Carbohydrate: 10.3g
- Fiber: 7.4g
- Protein: 7.6g
- Fat: 15.5g
- Sugar: 0.2g
- Sodium: 1mg

# Nuts & Seeds Bread

**(Yields:** 12 servings / **Prep Time:** 15 minutes / **Cooking Time:** 1 hour 10 minutes)

## Ingredients

- ½ cup raw pumpkin seeds
- ½ cup raw hazelnuts
- ½ cup raw almonds
- 1 cup raw sunflower seeds
- ½ cup chia seeds
- ½ cup golden flax seeds
- ½ cup psyllium husks
- ¼ cup golden flax seeds meal
- 1 teaspoon salt
- 1 teaspoon powdered stevia
- 3 tablespoons coconut oil, melted
- 1½ cups warm water

## Instructions

1. Preheat the oven to 350 degrees F. Line a bread loaf pan with a parchment paper.
2. Add the pumpkin seeds, hazelnuts and almonds in a food processor and pulse until a coarse flour like mixture is formed.
3. Add the nuts mixture, sunflower seeds, chia seeds, flax seeds, psyllium husks, flax seeds meal, salt, powder stevia, coconut oil and warm water in a large bowl and mix until well combined.
4. Place the mixture into prepared bread loaf pan and with your hands, press firmly to smooth the top surface.
5. Bake for about 45 minutes.
6. Carefully, transfer the bread loaf onto a baking sheet alongside the parchment paper.
7. Bake for about 15-25 minutes or until a toothpick inserted in the center comes out clean.
8. Remove the baking sheet from oven and place onto a wire rack to cool for about 15 minutes.
9. Carefully, invert the bread onto wire rack to cool completely before slicing.
10. With a sharp knife, cut the bread loaf into desired size slices and serve.

## Nutrition Values (Per Serving)

- Calories: 207
- Net Carbs: 2.7g
- Carbohydrate: 11.5g
- Fiber: 8.8g
- Protein: 7g
- Fat: 16.8g
- Sugar: 0.5g
- Sodium: 201mg

# Fresh Veggie Salad

**(Yields:** 4 servings / **Prep Time:** 20 minutes)

## Ingredients

- 2 cups cucumber, spiralized with blade C
- 1 cup Kalamata olives, pitted and halved
- 2 cups grape tomatoes, halved
- 1 tablespoon fresh oregano, chopped
- 1 tablespoon fresh basil, chopped
- 1 garlic clove, minced
- 2 tablespoons olive oil
- 2 tablespoons balsamic vinegar
- Salt and ground black pepper, as required

## Instructions

1. Place all the ingredients in a large serving bowl and toss to coat well.
2. Serve immediately.

## Nutrition Values (Per Serving)

- Calories: 129
- Net Carbs: 5.7g
- Carbohydrate: 8.6g
- Fiber: 2.9g
- Protein: 1.6g
- Fat: 11g
- Sugar: 3.3g
- Sodium: 338mg

---

# Lettuce Wraps

**(Yields:** 3 servings / **Prep Time:** 15 minutes)

## Ingredients

- ¾ cup fresh spinach, thinly sliced
- ½ of avocado, peeled, pitted and chopped
- ¾ cup cucumber, chopped
- 2 tablespoons scallions, chopped
- Salt and ground black pepper, as required
- 6 large lettuce leaves, rinsed and pat dried

## Instructions

1. Add the spinach, avocado, cucumber, scallion, salt and black pepper in a large bowl and mix well.
2. Arrange the lettuce leaves onto a smooth surface.
3. Divide the avocado mixture evenly onto each lettuce leaf.
4. Serve immediately.

### Nutrition Values (Per Serving)

- Calories: 77
- Net Carbs: 2g
- Carbohydrate: 4.7g
- Fiber: 2.7g
- Protein: 1.1g
- Fat: 6.6g
- Sugar: 0.8g
- Sodium: 60mg

---

## Pesto Zucchini Noodles

**(Yields:** 6 servings / **Prep Time:** 15 minutes)

### Ingredients

- 3 cups fresh spinach
- 4 garlic cloves, peeled
- ¼ cup raw pumpkin seeds
- 3 tablespoons oil
- Salt, as required
- 4 large zucchinis, spiralized with Blade C

### Instructions

1. Add all the ingredients except zucchini noodles in a blender and pulse until smooth.
2. Place the zucchini noodles and pesto in a large serving bowl and mix well.
3. Serve immediately.

### Nutrition Values (Per Serving)

- Calories: 132
- Net Carbs: 6g
- Carbohydrate: 9.1g
- Fiber: 3.1g
- Protein: 4.6g
- Fat: 10.1g
- Sugar: 3.9g
- Sodium: 62mg

---

## Roasted Broccoli & Cauliflower

**(Yields:** 8 servings / **Prep Time:** 15 minutes / **Cooking Time:** 20 minutes)

### Ingredients

- 4 cups cauliflower florets
- 4 cups broccoli florets
- 8 small garlic cloves, peeled and halved
- 2 tablespoons olive oil
- 2 tablespoons fresh lemon juice
- 1 teaspoon dried thyme, crushed
- 1 teaspoon dried oregano, crushed
- 1 teaspoon red pepper flakes, crushed
- Salt and ground black pepper, as required

## Instructions

1. Preheat the oven to 425 degrees F. Generously, grease 2 large baking dishes.
2. Add all the ingredients in a large bowl and toss to coat well.
3. Divide the vegetables into prepared baking dishes and spread in a single layer.
4. Roast for about 15-20 minutes or until the desired doneness of vegetables, tossing twice.
5. Remove from the oven and serve hot.

## Nutrition Values (Per Serving)

- Calories: 65
- Net Carbs: 4.4g
- Carbohydrate: 7.1g
- Fiber: 2.7g
- Protein: 2.5g
- Fat: 3.8g
- Sugar: 2.1g
- Sodium: 51mg

---

# Mushroom Stew

**(Yields:** 4 servings / **Prep Time:** 15 minutes / **Total Cooking Time:** 20 minutes)

## Ingredients

- 2 tablespoons olive oil
- 1 small yellow onions, chopped
- 2 garlic cloves, minced
- ½ pound fresh button mushrooms, sliced
- ¼ pound fresh shiitake mushrooms, sliced
- ¼ pound fresh Portobello mushrooms, sliced
- Salt and ground black pepper, as required
- ½ cup unsweetened coconut milk
- ¼ cup homemade vegetable broth
- 2 tablespoons fresh lemon juice
- 1 tablespoon fresh parsley, chopped

## Instructions

1. Heat the oil in a large skillet over medium heat and sauté the onion and garlic for about 5 minutes.
2. Stir in the mushrooms, salt, and black pepper and cook for about 5-7 minutes or until all the liquid is absorbed.
3. Stir in the coconut milk, and broth and bring to a gentle boil.
4. Simmer for about 5 minutes or until the desired doneness.
5. Stir in lemon juice and parsley and remove from the heat.
6. Serve hot.

### Nutrition Values (Per Serving)

- Calories: 102
- Net Carbs: 4.7g
- Carbohydrate: 6.4g
- Fiber: 1.7g
- Protein: 4.2g
- Fat: 7.8g
- Sugar: 2.9g
- Sodium: 96mg

---

## Cinnamon Ice Cream

**(Yields:** 5 servings / **Prep Time:** 15 minutes)

### Ingredients

- 1 tablespoon unsweetened gelatin powder*
- 1 tablespoon cold water
- 2 tablespoons hot water
- 27 ounces canned unsweetened coconut milk
- 1 tablespoon MCT oil
- 2 teaspoons ground cinnamon
- 2 teaspoons cinnamon liquid stevia
- 1 teaspoon organic vanilla extract
- Pinch of salt

### Instructions

1. Add the gelatin powder and cold water in a small bowl and mix well.
2. Now, add the hot water and mix until gelatin powder is dissolved completely.
3. Add the coconut milk, MCT oil, cinnamon, stevia, vanilla extract and salt in a high-speed blender and pulse on high speed until smooth.
4. Add the gelatin mixture and pulse on high speed until smooth.
5. Transfer the mixture into an ice cream maker and process according to the manufacturer's instructions.
6. Now, transfer the ice cream into an airtight container and freeze for at least 1-2 hours before serving.

### Nutrition Values (Per Serving)

- Calories: 288
- Net Carbs: 7g
- Carbohydrate: 8g
- Fiber: 1g
- Protein: 3.5g
- Fat: 28.3g
- Sugar: 2.7g
- Sodium: 97mg

(**Note: Gelatin powder** – Gelatin powder is not consider as vegan)

# Chocolate Tofu Mousse

**(Yields:** 4 servings / **Prep Time:** 15 minutes)

## Ingredients

- 1 pound firm tofu, pressed and drained
- 2 tablespoons cacao powder
- ¼ cup unsweetened almond milk
- 10 drops liquid stevia
- 1 tablespoon organic vanilla extract

## Instructions

1. Add all the ingredients in a blender and pulse until creamy and smooth.
2. Transfer the mousse into 4 serving bowls.
3. Refrigerate to chill for at least 2 hours before serving.

## Nutrition Values (Per Serving)

- Calories: 97
- Net Carbs: 1.9g
- Carbohydrate: 3.7g
- Fiber: 1.8g
- Protein: 9.9g
- Fat: 5.5g
- Sugar: 1.1g
- Sodium: 25mg

---

# Blueberry Scones

**(Yields:** 8 servings / **Prep Time:** 20 minutes / **Cooking Time:** 22 minutes)

## Ingredients

**For Scones:**
- 1 tablespoon ground flax seeds
- 3 tablespoons water
- 1 cup blanched almond flour
- ¼ cup coconut flour
- 3 tablespoons granulated Erythritol
- ½ teaspoon organic baking powder
- Salt, as required
- ¼ cup unsweetened almond milk
- 2 tablespoons coconut oil, melted
- 1 teaspoon organic vanilla extract
- ½ cup fresh blueberries

**For Glaze:**
- 2 tablespoons fresh blueberries
- 1 tablespoon coconut oil, melted
- 1 teaspoon granulated Erythritol

## Instructions

1. Preheat the oven to 350 degrees F. Line a baking sheet with a parchment paper.
2. For scones: add the ground flax seeds and water in a large bowl and mix until seeds are absorbed completely.

3. Set aside for about 5 minutes.
4. Add the flours, Erythritol, baking powder and salt in a bowl and mix until well combined.
5. In the bowl of flax seeds mixture, add the almond milk, coconut oil, and vanilla extract and beat until well combined.
6. Add the flour mixture and mix until a pliable dough forms.
7. Gently, fold in the blueberries.
8. Arrange the dough onto prepared baking sheet and with your hands, pat into about 1-inch thick circle.
9. Carefully, cut the circle into 8 equal-sized wedges.
10. Now, arrange the scones in a single layer about 1-inch apart.
11. Bake for about 18-22 minutes or until the top becomes golden brown.
12. Meanwhile, for the glaze: add all the ingredients in a blender and pulse until finely pureed.
13. Through a fine mesh sieve, strain the mixture and discard the blueberry skins.
14. Remove from oven and place the baking sheet onto a wire rack.
15. Spread the glaze evenly over each scone and let it cool completely before serving.

## Nutrition Values (Per Serving)

- Calories: 157
- Net Carbs: 4.1g
- Carbohydrate: 7.7g
- Fiber: 3.6g
- Protein: 3.8g
- Fat: 12.6g
- Sugar: 1.2g
- Sodium: 31mg

---

# Pumpkin Pudding

**(Yields:** 6 servings / **Prep Time:** 15 minutes / **Cooking Time:** 3 minutes)

## Ingredients

**For Pudding:**
- ¼ cup lukewarm water
- 1 (14-ounces) can unsweetened coconut milk
- 1 tablespoon unflavored gelatin powder*
- 1 (14-ounces) can organic pumpkin
- 2 tablespoons Erythritol
- 2 teaspoons organic vanilla extract
- 1/8 teaspoon liquid stevia
- 1 teaspoon ground cinnamon
- ¼ teaspoon ground ginger
- 1/8 teaspoon ground cloves
- Salt, as required

**For Topping:**
- ½ cup coconut cream
- 1 tablespoon powdered Erythritol
- ½ teaspoon ground cinnamon

## Instructions

1. Add the warm water and gelatin powder in a pan and stir until well combined.
2. Set aside for about 5 minutes.
3. Meanwhile, add the coconut milk, pumpkin, Erythritol, vanilla extract, stevia, spices and salt in a pan and cook for about 2-3 minutes or until just warmed.
4. Remove from the heat.
5. Add the gelatin mixture and beat until well combined and smooth.
6. Transfer the pudding into serving bowls.
7. With 1 plastic wrap, cover each bowl and refrigerate until set completely.
8. Meanwhile, for the topping: in a bowl, add all the ingredients and beat until soft peaks form.
9. Top each pudding cup with the whipped coconut cream and serve.

## Nutrition Values (Per Serving)

- Calories: 207
- Net Carbs: 6.8g
- Carbohydrate: 10.5g
- Fiber: 3.7g
- Protein: 4.3g
- Fat: 17.7g
- Sugar: 4g
- Sodium: 45mg

**(Note: Gelatin powder** – Gelatin powder is not consider as vegan**)**

# Measurements Conversion Charts

The charts you are seeing below will help you to convert the difference between units of volume in US customary units.

Please note that US volume is not the same as in the UK and other countries, and many of the measurements are different depending on your country.

It's very easy to get confused when dealing with US and UK units. The good thing is that the metric units never change.

All the measurement charts below are for US customary units only.

We have gone to great length in order to make sure that the measurements are on the following Measurement Charts are accurate.

| Term | Abbreviation | Nationality | Dry or liquid | Metric equivalent | Equivalent in context |
|---|---|---|---|---|---|
| **cup** | c., C. | | usually liquid | 237 milliliters | 16 tablespoons or 8 ounces |
| **ounce** | fl oz, fl. oz. | American | liquid only | 29.57 milliliters | |
| | | British | either | 28.41 milliliters | |
| **gallon** | gal. | American | liquid only | 3.785 liters | 4 quarts |
| | | British | either | 4.546 liters | 4 quarts |
| **inch** | in, in. | | | 2.54 centimeters | |
| **ounce** | oz, oz. | American | dry | 28.35 grams | 1/16 pound |
| | | | liquid | see OUNCE | see OUNCE |
| **pint** | p., pt. | American | liquid | 0.473 liter | 1/8 gallon or 16 ounces |
| | | | dry | 0.551 liter | 1/2 quart |
| | | British | either | 0.568 liter | |
| **pound** | lb. | | dry | 453.592 grams | 16 ounces |
| **Quart** | q., qt, qt. | American | liquid | 0.946 liter | 1/4 gallon or 32 ounces |
| | | | dry | 1.101 liters | 2 pints |
| | | British | either | 1.136 liters | |
| **Teaspoon** | t., tsp., tsp | | either | about 5 milliliters | 1/3 tablespoon |
| **Tablespoon** | T., tbs., tbsp. | | either | about 15 milliliters | 3 teaspoons or 1/2 ounce |

American and British Variances

## Volume (Liquid)

| American Standard (Cups & Quarts) | American Standard (Ounces) | Metric (Milliliters & Liters) |
|---|---|---|
| 2 tbsp. | 1 fl. oz. | 30 ml |
| 1/4 cup | 2 fl. oz. | 60 ml |
| 1/2 cup | 4 fl. oz. | 125 ml |
| 1 cup | 8 fl. oz. | 250 ml |
| 1 1/2 cups | 12 fl. oz. | 375 ml |
| 2 cups or 1 pint | 16 fl. oz. | 500 ml |
| 4 cups or 1 quart | 32 fl. oz. | 1000 ml or 1 liter |
| 1 gallon | 128 fl. oz. | 4 liters |

## Volume (Dry)

| American Standard | Metric |
|---|---|
| 1/8 teaspoon | 5 ml |
| 1/4 teaspoon | 1 ml |
| 1/2 teaspoon | 2 ml |
| 3/4 teaspoon | 4 ml |
| 1 teaspoon | 5 ml |
| 1 tablespoon | 15 ml |
| 1/4 cup | 59 ml |
| 1/3 cup | 79 ml |
| 1/2 cup | 118 ml |
| 2/3 cup | 158 ml |
| 3/4 cup | 177 ml |
| 1 cup | 225 ml |
| 2 cups or 1 pint | 450 ml |
| 3 cups | 675 ml |
| 4 cups or 1 quart | 1 liter |
| 1/2 gallon | 2 liters |
| 1 gallon | 4 liters |

## Oven Temperatures

| American Standard | Metric |
|---|---|
| 250° F | 130° C |
| 300° F | 150° C |
| 350° F | 180° C |
| 400° F | 200° C |
| 450° F | 230° C |

## Weight (Mass)

| American Standard (Ounces) | Metric (Grams) |
|---|---|
| 1/2 ounce | 15 grams |
| 1 ounce | 30 grams |
| 3 ounces | 85 grams |
| 3.75 ounces | 100 grams |
| 4 ounces | 115 grams |
| 8 ounces | 225 grams |
| 12 ounces | 340 grams |
| 16 ounces or 1 pound | 450 grams |

## Dry Measure Equivalents

| | | | |
|---|---|---|---|
| 3 teaspoons | 1 tablespoon | 1/2 ounce | 14.3 grams |
| 2 tablespoons | 1/8 cup | 1 ounce | 28.3 grams |
| 4 tablespoons | 1/4 cup | 2 ounces | 56.7 grams |
| 5 1/3 tablespoons | 1/3 cup | 2.6 ounces | 75.6 grams |
| 8 tablespoons | 1/2 cup | 4 ounces | 113.4 grams |
| 12 tablespoons | 3/4 cup | 6 ounces | .375 pound |
| 32 tablespoons | 2 cups | 16 ounces | 1 pound |

# About the Author

As one of seven children, Rachel Collins grew up in Cleveland, Ohio before moving to the mountains of Colorado in her early teens. From a young age she dreamed of moving to LA and becoming a fashion stylist. But when Rachel was fifteen, her only sister was born. Ever determined to rein in the chaos of her big family and have dinner on the table before midnight. Rachel began doing the cooking. She eventually discovered a new found freedom and a creativity she hadn't known existed. She began chronicling her fresh takes on old favorites and coupling them with her styling skills - only this time on tables and cutting boards - on her blog.

Since then, lots of people have fallen in love with her unique recipes, stunning photography, and charming life in her barn, which she has made into her home, high up in the snow-capped mountains.

Finally, before you go, I'd like to say "thank you" for purchasing my book and I hope that you had as much fun reading it as I had writing it.

I know you could have picked from dozens of books on keto diet recipes, but you took a chance with my guide. So, big thanks for purchasing this book and reading all the way to the end.

Now, I'd like to ask for a *small* favor. Could you please take a minute or two and leave a review for this book on Amazon by returning to your order history, the top right-hand side of your screen.

This feedback will help me continue to write the kind of books that will help you get results and help me to compete with other big publishers and authors.

**I bid you farewell and encourage you to move forward and find your true ketogenic diet spirit!**

Thank you and good luck!

—Rachel Collins

# RECIPE INDEX

## A

Almond
- Almond Brittles, 166
- Almond Butter, 255

Asparagus
- Bacon Wrapped Asparagus, 147
- Buttered Asparagus, 214
- Shrimp with Asparagus, 184

Avocado
- Avocado & Spinach Smoothie, 19
- Avocado Cups, 35
- Avocado Salsa, 155
- Avocado Sauce, 245
- Chicken Stuffed Avocado, 133
- Chilled Avocado Soup, 36

## B

Baba
- Baba Ghanoush, 248

Bacon
- Bacon & Jalapeño Soup, 43
- Bacon Omelet, 31
- Bacon Wrapped Asparagus, 147
- Bacon Wrapped Chicken Breast, 132
- Bacon Wrapped Pork Tenderloin, 109
- Bacon Wrapped Salmon, 173
- Bacon Wrapped Scallops, 154
- Bacon Wrapped Turkey Breast, 140
- Zucchini & Bacon Hash, 34

Basil
- Basil Pesto, 246
- Basil Pork Chops, 106
- Tomato & Basil Soup, 39

BBQ
- BBQ Sauce, 251

Beans
- Curried Broccoli, 207
- Shrimp & Green Beans Salad, 55

Beef
- Beef & Cabbage Stew, 64
- Beef & Mushroom Chili, 65
- Beef & Mushroom Soup, 47
- Beef & Zucchini Lasagna, 75
- Beef Burgers with Yogurt Sauce, 76
- Beef Casserole, 71
- Beef Crust Pizza, 73
- Beef Curry, 62
- Beef Muffins, 29
- Beef Salad, 59
- Beef Stew, 63
- Beef Stuffed Bell Peppers, 74
- Beef Taco Bake, 70
- Beef Taco Soup, 48
- Beef with Mushroom Gravy, 66

Bell Peppers
- Bell Pepper with Yellow Squash, 209
- Stuffed Bell Peppers, 208

Berries
- Berries & Spinach Salad, 51
- Mixed Berries Smoothie, 16

Biscuits
- Cheddar Biscuits, 161

Blackberry
- Blackberry Cobbler, 225
- Blackberry Smoothie, 14

Blueberry
- Blueberry & Lettuce Smoothie, 16
- Blueberry Bread, 29
- Blueberry Scones, 267
- Blueberry Smoothie, 15
- Mini Blueberry Bites, 163
- Steak with Blueberry Sauce, 67
- Tenderloin with Blueberry Sauce, 99

Bread
- Cheddar Bread, 30
- Nuts & Seeds Bread, 262

Breast
- Creamy Turkey Breast, 139
- Grilled Turkey Breast, 139

Broccoli
- Broccoli Casserole, 194
- Broccoli Mash, 216
- Broccoli Salad, 53
- Broccoli Soup, 42
- Broccoli Tots, 145
- Chicken & Broccoli Bake, 127
- Curried Broccoli, 207
- Garlicky Broccoli, 213
- Roasted Broccoli & Cauliflower, 264
- Scallops with Broccoli, 187

Brussels Sprout
- Brussels Sprout Chips, 158
- Creamy Brussels Sprout, 204
- Lemony Brussels Sprout, 213
- Pork with Brussels Sprout, 95

Buffalo
- Buffalo Chicken Bites, 151
- Chicken in Cheesy Buffalo Sauce, 123

Burgers
- Feta Turkey Burgers, 142
- Grilled Lamb Burgers, 79

Butter
- Almond Butter, 255
- Butter Chicken, 121
- Butter Coffee, 229
- Buttered Asparagus, 214
- Buttered Crepes, 27
- Buttered Pork Chops, 107
- Buttered Scallops, 188

Buttered Turkey Drumsticks, 141
Buttered Yellow Squash Noodles, 212
Cod in Butter Sauce, 176

# C

Cabbage
Beef & Cabbage Stew, 64
Braised Cabbage, 210
Cabbage Casserole, 192
Cabbage Salad, 51
Lamb with Cabbage, 78

Caesar Dressing, 239

Capers
Herbed Capers Sauce, 246

Catfish Stew, 169

Cauliflower
Cauliflower & Cottage Cheese Curry, 205
Cauliflower Casserole, 193
Cauliflower Mash, 215
Cauliflower Popcorns, 158
Cauliflower Soup, 41
Roasted Broccoli & Cauliflower, 264

Cereal
Mocha Cereal, 261

Cheddar
Cheddar Biscuits, 161
Cheddar Bread, 30
Cheddar Waffles, 24

Cheese
3 Cheese Crackers, 159
Blue Cheese Dressing, 240
Cheese & Olives Pizza, 196
Cheese Balls, 150
Cheese Bites, 160
Cheese Chips, 160
Cheese Crepes, 26
Cheesy Cauliflower, 204
Cheesy Pork Cutlets, 104
Cheesy Salmon, 170
Cheesy Tilapia, 178
Cheesy Tomato Slices, 146
Meatballs in Cheese Sauce, 89
No-Bake Cheesecake, 226
Spinach in Cheese Sauce, 203
Steak with Cheese Sauce, 67

Chicken
Bacon Wrapped Chicken Breast, 132
Buffalo Chicken Bites, 151
Butter Chicken, 121
Cheesy Chicken Soup, 44
Chicken & Broccoli Bake, 127
Chicken & Cauliflower Soup, 45
Chicken & Mushroom Soup, 46
Chicken & Salsa Soup, 44
Chicken & Veggie Bake, 128
Chicken Chili, 120
Chicken Cordon Bleu, 130
Chicken Frittata, 33
Chicken in Capers Sauce, 123
Chicken in Cheesy Buffalo Sauce, 123
Chicken in Creamy Spinach Sauce, 124
Chicken Kabobs, 133
Chicken Nuggets, 156
Chicken Parmigiana, 129
Chicken Popcorns, 155
Chicken Salad, 61
Chicken Stuffed Avocado, 133
Chicken with Zucchini Pasta, 125
Creamy Chicken Casserole, 126
Glazed Chicken Thighs, 118
Grilled Whole Chicken, 114
Parmesan Chicken Drumsticks, 117
Parmesan Chicken Wings, 150
Roasted Spatchcock Chicken, 115
Roasted Whole Chicken, 114
Spicy Chicken Curry, 122
Spicy Chicken Leg Quarters, 119
Stuffed Chicken Thighs, 131
Tangy Chicken Breasts, 119

Chili
Beef & Mushroom Chili, 65
Pork & Chiles Stew, 91
Turkey & Veggie Chili, 135

Chips
Brussels Sprout Chips, 158

Chives Scramble, 32

Chocolate
Chai Hot Chocolate, 229
Chocolate Chili, 90
Chocolate Coconut Bars, 164
Chocolate Fat Bombs, 163
Chocolate Lava Cake, 227
Chocolate Panna Cota, 222
Chocolate Pudding, 219
Chocolate Smoothie, 17
Chocolate Tofu Mousse, 267
Chocolaty Veggie Smoothie, 20
Hot Chocolate, 228

Chops
Baked Lamb Chops, 84
Basil Pork Chops, 106
Broiled Lamb Chops, 83
Buttered Pork Chops, 107
Lamb Chops with Cream Sauce, 81
Lamb Chops with Garlic Sauce, 80
Parmesan Pork Chops, 105
Spiced Pork Chops, 107
Stuffed Pork Chops, 108
Sweet & Sour Pork Chops, 104

Cilantro
Cilantro Sauce, 245
Fried Pork & Cilantro, 94

Cinnamon
Cinnamon Cappuccino, 230
Cinnamon Cookies, 162
Cinnamon Ice Cream, 266

Clams
Steamed Clams, 189

Cobbler
Blackberry Cobbler, 225

Coconut
Coconut Cereal, 22
Coconut Shrimp, 153
Coconut Tilapia, 178

Cod
Cod & Vegetables Bake, 175
Cod in Butter Sauce, 176

Coffee
- Butter Coffee, 229
- Coffee Granita, 217
- Espresso Coffee, 230
- Iced Coffee, 237

Cornish
- Stuffed Cornish Hens, 116

Crab
- Crab Salad, 58
- Lemony Crab Legs, 190

Cranberry Sauce, 243

Cream
- Cream Cake, 227
- Cream Cheese Flan, 223
- Cream Cheese Muffins, 28
- Cream Cheese Pancake, 25
- Cream Cheese Salmon, 170
- Cream Fudge, 223
- Cream Tartlets, 224
- Creamy Brussels Sprout, 204
- Creamy Ground Turkey, 134
- Creamy Iced Tea, 236
- Creamy Mustard Dressing, 241
- Creamy Pork Loin, 101
- Creamy Porridge, 22
- Creamy Shrimp Salad, 55
- Creamy Turkey Breast, 139
- Creamy Zucchini Noodles, 211
- Prawns in Creamy Mushroom Sauce, 186
- Shrimp in Cream Sauce, 182
- Vanilla Crème Brûlée, 220

Crepes
- Buttered Crepes, 27

Croquettes
- Tuna Croquettes, 157

Cucumber
- Chilled Cucumber Soup, 36
- Cucumber & Parsley Smoothie, 18
- Cucumber & Spinach Salad, 52
- Cucumber Cups, 143

Curry
- Beef Curry, 62
- Curried Broccoli, 207
- Curried Veggies Bake, 200
- Curry Powder, 259
- Eggplant Curry, 206
- Grouper & Tomato Curry, 167
- Lamb Curry, 77
- Meatballs Curry, 88
- Salmon Curry, 168
- Shrimp Curry, 185
- Spicy Steak Curry, 63

Custard
- Mascarpone Custard, 219

## D

Drumsticks
- Buttered Turkey Drumsticks, 141
- Parmesan Chicken Drumsticks, 117

## E

Egg
- Deviled Eggs, 143
- Eggnog, 233

Eggplant
- Eggplant Curry, 206
- Eggplant Lasagna, 195

Enchilada Sauce, 252

Espresso Coffee, 230

## F

Fat
- Chocolate Fat Bombs, 163

Feta
- Feta Turkey Burgers, 142
- Olives & Feta Dressing, 241

Flan
- Cream Cheese Flan, 223

French Dressing, 238

Fried
- Pan Fried Squid, 187

Fried Pork & Cilantro, 94

Frittata
- Chicken Frittata, 33

Fruit & Veggies Smoothie, 20

Fudge
- Cream Fudge, 223

## G

Garlic
- Garlicky Broccoli, 213
- Garlicky Haddock, 177
- Garlicky Pork Shoulder, 97
- Garlicky Prime Rib Roast, 70
- Lamb Chops with Garlic Sauce, 80
- Scallops in Garlic Sauce, 189

Ghanoush
- Baba Ghanoush, 248

Ginger
- Ginger Lemonade, 235
- Gingerbread Latte, 231

Granita
- Coffee Granita, 217

Granola
- Seeds Granola, 21

Green
- Green Veggies Smoothie, 19
- Green Veggies Soup, 38
- Ground Pork with Greens, 110
- Lemony Green Tea, 233
- Mint Green Tea, 235
- Shrimp & Green Beans Salad, 55

Grilled Steak, 68

## H

Haddock
- Garlicky Haddock, 177

Halibut
- Parmesan Halibut, 176

Hash
- Zucchini & Bacon Hash, 34

Hens
- Stuffed Cornish Hens, 116

Herb
- Herbed Capers Sauce, 246
- Herbed Sardines, 181

Hoisin Sauce, 253

Hummus
- Veggie Hummus, 247

## I

Ice
- Cinnamon Ice Cream, 266
- Creamy Iced Tea, 236
- Iced Coffee, 237
- Mocha Ice Cream, 217

Italian Dressing, 242

## J

Jalapeño
- Bacon & Jalapeño Soup, 43
- Jalapeño Poppers, 148

Juice
- Fresh Strawberry Juice, 260

## K

Kabobs
- Chicken Kabobs, 133

Ketchup, 244

## L

Lamb
- Baked Lamb Chops, 84
- Broiled Lamb Chops, 83
- Grilled Lamb Burgers, 79
- Grilled Leg of Lamb, 85
- Grilled Rack of Lamb, 82
- Lamb Chops with Cream Sauce, 81
- Lamb Chops with Garlic Sauce, 80
- Lamb Curry, 77
- Lamb Stew, 76
- Lamb with Cabbage, 78
- Roasted Lamb Shanks, 80
- Roasted Leg of Lamb, 85
- Stuffed Leg of Lamb, 86

Lasagna
- Beef & Zucchini Lasagna, 75
- Eggplant Lasagna, 195

Lemon
- Ginger Lemonade, 235
- Lemon Soufflé, 221
- Lemonade, 234
- Lemony Brussels Sprout, 213
- Lemony Crab Legs, 190
- Lemony Green Tea, 233
- Lemony Trout, 181

Lettuce
- Blueberry & Lettuce Smoothie, 16
- Lettuce Wraps, 263

Liver
- Pork Liver with Scallion, 96

Loaf
- Veggie Loaf, 199

Lobster Salad, 57

Loin
- Creamy Pork Loin, 101
- Sweet & Tangy Pork Loin, 101

## M

Marinara Sauce, 251

Mascarpone Custard, 219

Mash
- Broccoli Mash, 216
- Cauliflower Mash, 215

Mayonnaise, 256

Meatball
- Meatballs Curry, 88
- Meatballs in Cheese Sauce, 89
- Meatballs Soup, 50

Meatloaf
- Pork & Spinach Meatloaf, 111

Mint Green Tea, 235

Mocha
- Mocha Cereal, 261
- Mocha Ice Cream, 217

Mousse
- Chocolate Tofu Mousse, 267

Mozzarella
- Mozzarella Sticks, 149
- Tomato & Mozzarella Salad, 53

Muffins
- Beef Muffins, 29
- Cream Cheese Muffins, 28

Mushroom
- Beef & Mushroom Chili, 65
- Beef & Mushroom Soup, 47
- Beef with Mushroom Gravy, 66
- Chicken & Mushroom Soup, 46
- Mini Mushroom Pizzas, 148
- Mushroom Soup, 41
- Mushroom Stew, 265
- Prawns in Creamy Mushroom Sauce, 186
- Spiced mushroom, 214

Mustard
- Creamy Mustard Dressing, 241

Mustard Pork Tenderloin, 100

## N

Noodle
- Buttered Yellow Squash Noodles, 212
- Creamy Zucchini Noodles, 211
- Pesto Zucchini Noodles, 264

Nuggets
- Chicken Nuggets, 156

Nut Crusted Salmon, 172

Nuts & Seeds Bread, 262

## O

Olive
- Cheese & Olives Pizza, 196
- Olives & Feta Dressing, 241

Omelet
- Bacon Omelet, 31

## P

Pan Fried Squid, 187

Pancake
- Cream Cheese Pancakes, 25
- Spinach Pancakes, 25

Panna
- Chocolate Panna Cota, 222

Parmesan
- Parmesan Chicken Drumsticks, 117
- Parmesan Chicken Wings, 150
- Parmesan Halibut, 176

Parmigiana
- Chicken Parmigiana, 129

Parsley
  Cucumber & Parsley Smoothie, 18
Pasta
  Chicken with Zucchini Pasta, 125
Pesto
  Basil Pesto, 246
Pesto Zucchini Noodles, 264
Pie
  Salmon Pie, 174
  Shepherd Pie, 72
  Spinach Pie, 198
Pizza
  Cheese & Olives Pizza, 196
  Mini Mushroom Pizzas, 148
  Pizza Sauce, 250
  Turkey Pizza, 137
  Zucchini Pizza, 197
Popcorns
  Cauliflower Popcorns, 158
  Chicken Popcorns, 155
Pork
  Bacon Wrapped Pork Tenderloin, 109
  Basil Pork Chops, 106
  Braised Pork Shoulder, 98
  Buttered Pork Chops, 107
  Cheesy Pork Cutlets, 104
  Creamy Pork Loin, 101
  Fried Pork & Cilantro, 94
  Garlicky Pork Shoulder, 97
  Ground Pork with Greens, 110
  Mustard Pork Tenderloin, 100
  Parmesan Pork Chops, 105
  Pork & Chiles Stew, 91
  Pork & Spinach Meatloaf, 111
  Pork Casserole, 113
  Pork Liver with Scallion, 96
  Pork Pinwheel, 112
  Pork Stew, 90
  Pork Stroganoff, 92
  Pork with Brussels Sprout, 95
  Pork with Sauerkraut, 93
  Pork with Veggies, 96
  Spiced Pork Chops, 107
  Spicy Baked Pork Ribs, 103
  Sticky Baked Pork Ribs, 102
  Stuffed Pork Chops, 108
  Stuffed Pork Tenderloin, 109
  Sweet & Sour Pork Chops, 104
  Sweet & Tangy Pork Loin, 101
Porridge
  Creamy Porridge, 22
  Overnight Porridge, 260
Poultry Seasoning, 257
Powder
  Curry Powder, 259
Prawns in Creamy Mushroom Sauce, 186
Protein
  Strawberry Protein Smoothie, 13
Pudding
  Chocolate Pudding, 219
Pumpkin
  Pumpkin Pie Spice, 258
  Pumpkin Porridge, 23
  Pumpkin Pudding, 268
  Pumpkin Smoothie, 18

**Q**

Quiche
  Spinach Quiche, 33

**R**

Ranch Dressing, 238
Raspberry
  Raspberry Dressing, 243
  Raspberry Smoothie, 14
Rib
  Garlicky Prime Rib Roast, 70

**S**

Salad
  Beef Salad, 59
  Berries & Spinach Salad, 51
  Broccoli Salad, 53
  Cabbage Salad, 51
  Chicken Salad, 61
  Crab Salad, 58
  Creamy Shrimp Salad, 55
  Cucumber & Spinach Salad, 52
  Fresh Veggie Salad, 263
  Lobster Salad, 57
  Mixed Veggie Salad, 54
  Salad Wraps, 210
  Salmon Salad, 56
  Shrimp & Green Beans Salad, 55
  Tomato & Mozzarella Salad, 53
  Tuna Salad, 58
  Turkey Salad, 60
Salmon
  Bacon Wrapped Salmon, 173
  Broiled Salmon, 171
  Cheesy Salmon, 170
  Cream Cheese Salmon, 170
  Mini Salmon Bites, 152
  Nut Crusted Salmon, 172
  Salmon Curry, 168
  Salmon Pie, 174
  Stuffed Salmon, 172
Salsa
  Avocado Salsa, 155
Salsa Verde, 249
Sardines
  Herbed Sardines, 181
Sauce
  Avocado Sauce, 245
  BBQ Sauce, 251
  Beef Burgers with Yogurt Sauce, 76
  Chicken in Capers Sauce, 123
  Chicken in Cheesy Buffalo Sauce, 123
  Chicken in Creamy Spinach Sauce, 124
  Cilantro Sauce, 245
  Cod in Butter Sauce, 176
  Cranberry Sauce, 243
  Enchilada Sauce, 252
  Herbed Capers Sauce, 246
  Hoisin Sauce, 253
  Hot Sauce, 254
  Lamb Chops with Cream Sauce, 81
  Lamb Chops with Garlic Sauce, 80

Marinara Sauce, 251
Meatballs in Cheese Sauce, 89
Pizza Sauce, 250
Prawns in Creamy Mushroom Sauce, 186
Tenderloin with Blueberry Sauce, 99
Teriyaki Sauce, 253
Worcestershire Sauce, 255

Sauerkraut
  Pork with Sauerkraut, 93
Scallion
  Pork Liver with Scallion, 96
Scallops
  Bacon Wrapped Scallops, 154
  Buttered Scallops, 188
  Scallops in Garlic Sauce, 189
  Scallops with Broccoli, 187
Scones
  Blueberry Scones, 267
Scramble
  Chives Scramble, 32
Seasoned Salt, 257
Seeds
  Nuts & Seeds Bread, 262
  Seeds Granola, 21
Shanks
  Roasted Lamb Shanks, 80
Shepherd Pie, 72
Shrimp
  Coconut Shrimp, 153
  Shrimp & Tomato Bake, 184
  Shrimp Curry, 185
  Shrimp in Cream Sauce, 182
  Shrimp with Asparagus, 184
  Shrimp with Zucchini, 183
Smoothie
  Avocado & Spinach Smoothie, 19
  Blackberry Smoothie, 14
  Blueberry & Lettuce Smoothie, 16
  Blueberry Smoothie, 15
  Chocolate Smoothie, 17
  Chocolaty Veggie Smoothie, 20
  Cucumber & Parsley Smoothie, 18
  Fruit & Veggies Smoothie, 20
  Green Veggies Smoothie, 19
  Mixed Berries Smoothie, 16
  Pumpkin Smoothie, 18
  Raspberry Smoothie, 14
  Vanilla Smoothie, 17
Soup
  Bacon & Jalapeño Soup, 43
  Beef & Mushroom Soup, 47
  Beef Taco Soup, 48
  Broccoli Soup, 42
  Cauliflower Soup, 41
  Cheesy Chicken Soup, 44
  Chicken & Cauliflower Soup, 45
  Chicken & Mushroom Soup, 46
  Chicken & Salsa Soup, 44
  Chilled Avocado Soup, 36
  Chilled Cucumber Soup, 36
  Chilled Strawberry Soup, 38
  Chilled Tomato Soup, 37
  Green Veggies Soup, 38
  Meatballs Soup, 50
  Mushroom Soup, 41
  Salmon Soup, 48
  Tilapia Soup, 49
  Tomato & Basil Soup, 39
  Yellow Squash Soup, 40
Spatchcock
  Roasted Spatchcock Chicken, 115
Spinach
  Berries & Spinach Salad, 51
  Chicken in Creamy Spinach Sauce, 124
  Pork & Spinach Meatloaf, 111
  Spinach in Cheese Sauce, 203
  Spinach Pancakes, 25
  Spinach Pie, 198
  Spinach Quiche, 33
Squash
  Bell Pepper with Yellow Squash, 209
  Buttered Yellow Squash Noodles, 212
  Yellow Squash Casserole, 193
Squid
  Pan Fried Squid, 187
Steak
  Grilled Steak, 68
  Spicy Steak Curry, 63
  Steak with Blueberry Sauce, 67
  Steak with Cheese Sauce, 67
Stew
  Beef & Cabbage Stew, 64
  Beef Stew, 63
  Catfish Stew, 169
  Lamb Stew, 76
  Mixed Veggies Stew, 201
  Mushroom Stew, 265
  Pork & Chiles Stew, 91
  Pork Stew, 90
  Seafood Stew, 191
  Tofu & Veggies Stew, 202
Strawberry
  Fresh Strawberry Juice, 260
  Strawberry Protein Smoothie, 13
  Strawberry Smoothie, 13
  Strawberry Sundae, 218
Strips
  Tilapia Strips, 153
Stroganoff
  Pork Stroganoff, 92
Sunflower Seeds Dressing, 242
Sweet & Sour Pork Chops, 104

# T

Taco
  Beef Taco Bake, 70
  Beef Taco Soup, 48
  Taco Seasoning, 258
Tartlets
  Cream Tartlets, 224
Tea
  Creamy Iced Tea, 236
  Lemony Green Tea, 233
  Mint Green Tea, 235
  Spiced Tea, 232

Tenderloin
- Bacon Wrapped Pork Tenderloin, 109
- Mustard Pork Tenderloin, 100
- Roasted Tenderloin, 69
- Stuffed Pork Tenderloin, 109
- Tenderloin with Blueberry Sauce, 99

Teriyaki Sauce, 253

Thighs
- Glazed Chicken Thighs, 118
- Stuffed Chicken Thighs, 131

Tilapia
- Cheesy Tilapia, 178
- Coconut Tilapia, 178
- Tilapia Soup, 49
- Tilapia Strips, 153

Tofu
- Chocolate Tofu Mousse, 267
- Tofu & Veggies Stew, 202

Tomato
- Cheesy Tomato Slices, 146
- Chilled Tomato Soup, 37
- Grouper & Tomato Curry, 167
- Shrimp & Tomato Bake, 184
- Stuffed Tomatoes, 146
- Tomato & Basil Soup, 39
- Tomato & Mozzarella Salad, 53

Tots
- Broccoli Tots, 145

Trout
- Lemony Trout, 181

Tuna
- Tuna Casserole, 179
- Tuna Croquettes, 157
- Tuna Salad, 58

Turkey
- Bacon Wrapped Turkey Breast, 140
- Buttered Turkey Drumsticks, 141
- Creamy Ground Turkey, 134
- Creamy Turkey Breast, 139
- Feta Turkey Burgers, 142
- Grilled Turkey Breast, 139
- Spicy Roasted Turkey, 138
- Turkey & Veggie Chili, 135
- Turkey Casserole, 136
- Turkey Pizza, 137
- Turkey Salad, 60

Tzatziki, 248

# V

Vanilla
- Vanilla Crème Brûlée, 220
- Vanilla Smoothie, 17

Veggies
- Chicken & Veggie Bake, 128
- Chocolaty Veggie Smoothie, 20
- Cod & Vegetables Bake, 175
- Curried Veggies Bake, 200
- Fresh Veggie Salad, 263
- Fruit & Veggies Smoothie, 20
- Green Veggies Smoothie, 19
- Green Veggies Soup, 38
- Mixed Veggie Combo, 202
- Mixed Veggie Salad, 54
- Mixed Veggies Stew, 201
- Pork with Veggies, 96
- Tofu & Veggies Stew, 202
- Turkey & Veggie Chili, 135
- Veggie Hummus, 247
- Veggie Loaf, 199

Verde
- Salsa Verde, 249

# W

Waffles
- Cheddar Waffles, 24

Walnut Bark, 165

Wings
- Parmesan Chicken Wings, 150

Worcestershire Sauce, 255

# Y

Yogurt
- Beef Burgers with Yogurt Sauce, 76
- Yogurt Dressing, 239

# Z

Zucchini
- Beef & Zucchini Lasagna, 75
- Chicken with Zucchini Pasta, 125
- Creamy Zucchini Noodles, 211
- Grilled Zucchini, 212
- Pesto Zucchini Noodles, 264
- Shrimp with Zucchini, 183
- Stuffed Zucchini, 207
- Zucchini & Bacon Hash, 34
- Zucchini Pizza, 197
- Zucchini Sticks, 144

# YOU MAY BE INTERESTED IN MY OTHER COOKBOOKS

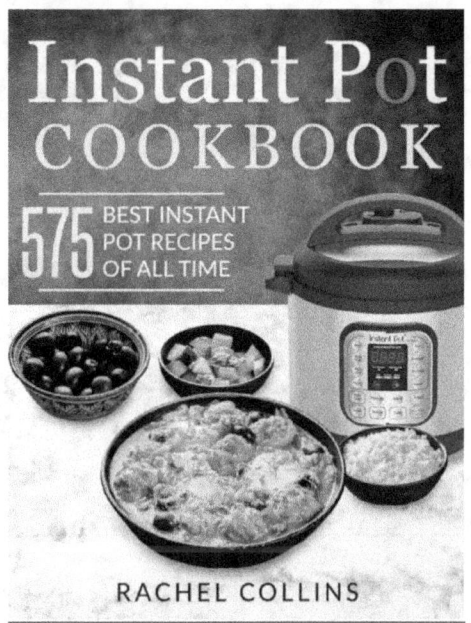

**Instant Pot Cookbook:
575 Best Instant Pot Recipes of All Time
(with Nutrition Facts, Easy and Healthy Recipes)**

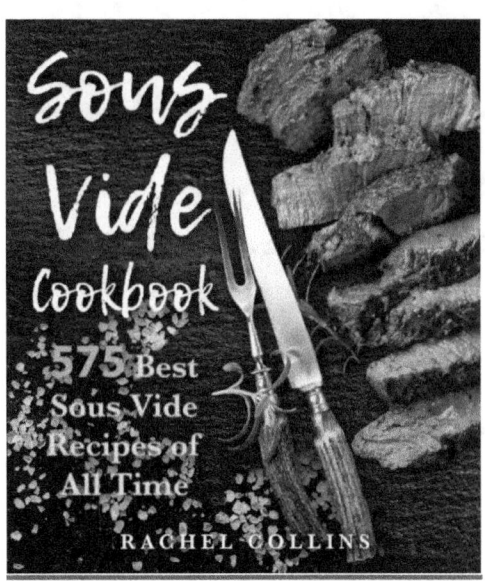

**Sous Vide Cookbook:
575 Best Sous Vide Recipes of All Time
(with Nutrition Facts and Everyday Recipes)**

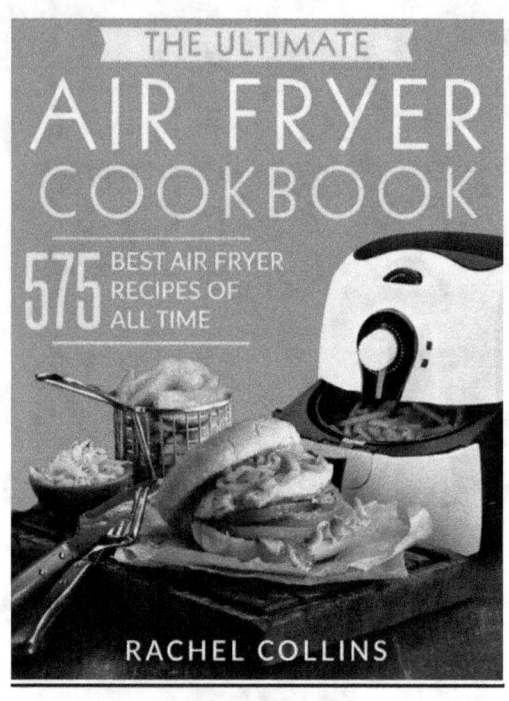

**The Ultimate Air Fryer Cookbook:
575 Best Air Fryer Recipes of All Time**

www.ingramcontent.com/pod-product-compliance
Lightning Source LLC
Chambersburg PA
CBHW051401070526
44584CB00023B/3247